RIPPED WITH BODYWEIGHT

12-Week Program for Muscle Growth and Fat Loss

Lane Goodwin

DISCLAIMER: You should consult your physician or other healthcare professional before starting this or any other fitness program to determine if it is right for your needs. This is particularly true if you (or your family) have a history of high blood pressure or heart disease, or if you have ever experienced chest pain when exercising or have experienced chest pain in the past month when not engaged in physical activity, smoke, have high cholesterol, are obese, or have a bone or joint problem that could be made worse by a change in physical activity. Do not start this fitness program if your physician or health care provider advises against it. If you experience faintness, dizziness, pain or shortness of breath at any time while exercising you should stop immediately.

This book offers health, fitness and nutritional information and is designed for educational purposes only. You should not rely on this information as a substitute for, nor does it replace professional medical advice, diagnosis, or treatment. If you have any concerns or questions about your health, you should always consult with a physician or other health-care professional. Do not disregard, avoid or delay obtaining medical or health related advice from your health-care professional because of something you may have read on this site. The use of any information provided on this book is solely at your own risk.

Developments in medical research may impact the health, fitness and nutritional advice that appears here. No assurance can be given that the advice contained in this book will always include the most recent findings or developments with respect to the particular material.

CONTENTS

INTRODUCTION

*Physical fitness is not only one of the most important
keys to a healthy body, it is the basis of dynamic
and creative intellectual activity*

—John F. Kennedy

Getting ripped had always been my dream but after a few failed attempts in my younger years, I had decided that it's not in my genetics to build muscle. I quietly accepted to be content with cardio (long distance running) and playing the occasional semi-weekly soccer match with my colleagues.

5 years ago, I moved to a new house which had a fancy gym nearby. Having this gym just 5 minutes walking distance away from my house rekindled the old flame of building muscle. I joined the gym, told them I wanted to build muscle and I was assigned a personal trainer to help me reach my goals.

My personal trainer wrote me a training schedule which I followed religiously to the letter for 6 months but I failed to build any muscle whatsoever. I quit the gym once again deciding that building muscle is not for me. Worse, I ate like a horse in these six months with the hopes of building muscle but I only managed to build fat. I was worse off after training for six months because not only had I failed to build muscle, but also I gained 10 extra pounds of fat that I had to get rid of. Once again, I had to reluctantly accept my inability to build muscle. I didn't know at the time but my savior would arrive soon.

It was the September of 2013 when one of my closest friends at the workplace was constantly talking about how he started high-intensity bodyweight training, and how much he liked it. I knew this man for years. He used to be a chubby, flabby guy although he used to do tons of cardio – just like me.

After a few weeks of training, his body started to change visibly. We used to wear t-shirts to work as we were software developers who didn't need to wear suits and it was easy to see that his arms and his chest were growing muscular. Everybody in the work-place was noticing his physical transformation and asking what the hell is he doing to grow this fast. Girls at the workplace were complimenting his physique.

On one of those days, we were getting our lunch in the company cafeteria. I still remember that day more vividly than yesterday. As we were standing in front of the counter, my friend was talk-ing about his previous evening's bodyweight training session. He was saying that some unbelievable things were happening to his muscles. He asked me to knock on his triceps muscles like I would knock on a door. I did, and I was instantly mindblown. It felt like I knocked on a concrete wall. It had only been about 4-weeks since he started bodyweight training and he already had arms of steel.

That day, I decided to start bodyweight training. My friend gave me his training routine and I was impatient until it's 5 p.m. and I could go home and do my first bodyweight workout. I imme-diately went home after work and did my training. It was tough and intense but I felt great. I had seen how much my friend im-proved in just a few weeks and I was determined to do the same. My muscles were sore the next day but I didn't care. In fact, I was happy. The muscles that I didn't even know to exist were sore and I knew in my heart that this was a good thing. I had never felt like this in my previous attempts to build muscle.

After a few weeks of training, I was getting similar results to my friend. My muscles quickly improved and I was getting compliments too from my coworkers, friends, and family. We were discussing our training sessions with my friend and sharing tips as we discover more efficient ways of training to improve our results. We were simplifying our training as we keep going and getting better results as we trained less and less. Before, I had never thought that I could get six-pack abs because I thought it was in the territory of fitness models and athletes. As my physique got better and better, I started to believe that I too can have six-pack abs.

I quit my job in January 2014 and moved to Thailand. I had solidified my bodyweight training routine and I could see my abs slightly showing but I needed to get leaner to uncover the ab muscles I built. I bought books and read blog posts about fat loss techniques but most of the published information was garbage. I wasted a lot of time with different kinds of inefficient diets until I found the diet that works and I finally got my six-pack abs. I rushed to a photo studio to immortalize the fact that I had six-pack abs, thinking that I might never have them again. Luckily, I later discovered that it's actually not difficult anymore for me to maintain my six-pack abs or get them back easily whenever I wanted to have them. I discovered that it's easy to maintain my muscle mass once I built them, thanks to a wonderful phenomenon called muscle memory.

I had meticulously noted down everything I ate during my quest for six-pack abs, so, it was easy for me to repeat the diet that allowed me to lose fat and uncover my six-pack abs. Having six-pack abs is a wonderful feeling, especially for an everyday man like me. I did it once and I will enjoy it for a lifetime.

The muscle building and fat burning wisdom I acquired during bodyweight training allow me to live my life without any worries about my fitness. When I gain a few pounds of fat, I know how to burn them. If I fail to train for a while and my muscles retreat, I can get them back in a few weeks. I learned how to build muscle and how to burn fat. This valuable knowledge will serve me for life. In this book, I will share that knowledge with you.

This book is the book I wish I had when I started building muscle. It's also the book I wish I had when I decided to get down to 8-10% of body fat. 99% of the muscle building and diet advice I found on the internet is garbage which is aimed to profit from the gullible people who want results without hard work.

The information you will find in this book is simple yet powerful. There are only a few exercises and a few dieting techniques and that's all. However, simple doesn't equal easy, mind you. Many people underestimate bodyweight training and think it's easy but that's only half true. The training routines in this book will require you to work hard. Building muscle isn't easy. Losing fat is fairly easier than building muscle but still, it's not easy.

Building muscle is achieved through resistance training. Bodyweight training is an excellent form of resistance training.

Burning fat is achieved mainly through diet. I made the mistake of thinking that training is enough to take care of fat loss but I paid dearly for my mistake. I learned the hard way that you can't out-train a bad diet. In this book, you will find the fat burning techniques to shred fat and the muscle building diet that will allow you to build muscle even when you are losing fat.

I am a busy person. I have businesses to run, loved ones to spend time with and a world to travel. I don't have enough time to train for long hours. I never train any longer than 3 hours per week. The training routines in this book will take you less than 3 hours per week on average too.

I picked the exercises that give you the most bang for your buck. All the exercises in this book are compound exercises which train multiple muscle groups at once. This saves you tremendous time compared to isolation exercises which train your muscle groups one by one.

Another benefit of the routines you will find in this book is that the time you spend training will decrease as you improve. With bodyweight training, less is more. For example, a man who can do 50 pushups in 30 seconds will have a better body than a man who can do the same number of push-ups in 10 minutes. Your aim should always be to shorten your training time. Within a short period of time, you will see that you are able to train more in 15 minutes than other people who waste hours on the treadmill. If doing 50 push-ups seems impossible to you at the moment, don't fret. Your body is an incredible machine. You will be surprised how quickly you will improve provided that you follow the instructions in this book.

To wrap up, here are the things you will find in this book:

- How to build a lean, strong and athletic body with bodyweight training by training less than 3 hours a week without any equipment other than a pull-up bar.
- Muscle building and fat burning diet methods to boost your muscle building efficiency, supercharge your metabolism to burn fat and uncover the six pack abs you will build by training.
- The 8 best bodyweight exercises for your arms, shoulders, back, chest, abs, glutes, and legs.
- The muscle building mindset to get the most out of your training.
- How to build the mental toughness to push through mental barriers.
- How to apply progressive overload to bodyweight training to make sure that your muscles are growing.
- Training guidelines to get the most out of your training.
- The benefits of strength training and bodyweight train-

ing.
- 12-week bodyweight training routines for beginner, intermediate, and advanced levels.

Don't keep your expectations low. If you follow the guidelines in this book, you can expect to get strong fast. I mean really fast.

Who Is This Book For

This book is for everybody who wants to have a lean, strong, and athletic body.

YOU DON'T HAVE THE TIME IN YOUR HANDS TO DEVOTE TO LONG HOURS OF TRAINING?

You will train less than 3 hours a week on average and your training time will decrease further as you progress.

YOU DON'T WANT TO SPEND YEARS WITH TRAINING UNTIL YOU GET THE LEAN, STRONG, AND ATHLETIC BODY YOU WANT?

The training routines and the diet techniques you'll find in this book are capable of providing fast results. You will notice your body changing visibly within a few weeks.

YOU ARE A BEGINNER AND YOU HAVE NO IDEA HOW TO TRAIN FOR STRENGTH?

The guidelines in the book are easy to follow, all the exercises have easier versions to get you started and I included a beginner routine for the ones who want to get their feet wet.

YOU CAN'T AFFORD A GYM?

You only need a pull-up bar or anything that allows you to do pull-ups and nothing else. You can do all your exercises in the comfort of your home, outside or anywhere else you want.

DO YOU THINK YOU ARE TOO OLD TO TRAIN FOR STRENGTH?

I started strength training at the age of 37, now I am 43 and I am stronger than ever. I keep breaking personal records. You can do it whatever your age is.

YOU CAN'T AFFORD SUPPLEMENTS OR SCARED THAT YOU WON'T GET RESULTS WITHOUT SUPPLEMENTS?

Supplements aren't necessary at all for enjoying the full benefits of this book.

YOU DON'T HAVE ANY ATHLETIC SKILLS?

Athletic skills are built through training, repetition, and consistency. There are enough reps within the training routines in this book. You will build athletic skills if you do the workouts.

ARE YOU ALREADY ENGAGING IN OTHER TYPES OF SPORTS?

Building muscle will improve your performance in any other sports you are doing. By doing the exercises in this book, you will run faster, jump higher, kick and throw the ball harder. Bodyweight training will take your strength and endurance to the next level.

DO YOU TRAVEL A LOT?

You can do many of the workouts in a hotel room and when your workout requires you to do pull-ups, anywhere you can do pull-ups is a good place to train.

CHAPTER 1: 10 REASONS WHY STRENGTH TRAINING IS SUPERIOR TO OTHER TYPES OF EXERCISE

*A truly strong person does not need the approval of others
any more than a lion needs the approval of sheep.*
—Vernon Howard

To be honest, I got into strength training to get a lean, strong and muscular body. It was only after I built the body I dreamed of that I started to realize that the benefits of strength training go a lot further than having a body that looks good.

The decision I made years ago to start bodyweight training still keeps providing incredible benefits to me and will continue to do so as long as I exert the minimum effort to maintain my physique.

Here are the benefits you can expect to enjoy from strength training:

1. Strength Training Helps You Burn Fat Even When You Are Sedentary

When you do cardio, you only burn calories during the exercise.

The moment you finish your workout is the moment you stop burning calories. Strength training builds muscle. Muscles are fat burning machines. Your muscles will burn calories 7 days 24 hours. As a result, it will be easier for you to lose fat whenever the circumstances require you to do so.

2. Strength Training Increases Testosterone

Testosterone is responsible for your muscular mass, cognitive functioning, sex drive, cardiovascular health, bone strength, confidence, and your overall well-being. Strength training is proven to increase testosterone, especially when you train your whole body, which you can achieve by doing the exercises in this book.

3. Strength Training Develops Every Muscle In Your Body

Whatever other sport you engage in, there will be some muscles more involved than the others. For example, when you play soccer, your leg muscles will work more than your other muscles. When you play tennis, your legs and forearms will develop but the rest of your muscles will not be significantly involved in your movements. In contrast, a full body strength training routine will work all the muscles in your body.

4. Strength Training Builds You An Attractive Body

Every fitness or beauty product ad will showcase a model with six-pack abs. This is no accident. A set of six-pack abs is the ultimate indicator of fitness. Six-pack abs don't pop up in a weak body. A visible set of six-pack abs is the indicator of a strong, lean, agile, coordinated and resilient body. You don't even have to look at the modern fitness ads to notice that a muscular male body is attractive. Look at the ancient Greek statues. All the Greek statues depict muscular men with six-pack abs. A muscular body is the timeless representative of an attractive male body.

5. Strength Training Fights Aging

One of the most visible indicators of aging is muscle loss and the weakening of the bones. Old people look frail because humans begin to gradually lose muscle mass and bone density after the age of 30. Most of the older age health problems are directly caused by loss of muscle and bone density. Strength training solves this problem by strengthening the muscles and the bones. Moreover, stronger muscles and bones decrease sagging, reduce wrinkles on the skin, improve posture, which help older people look younger and better.

6. Strength Training Prevents Cancer And Cardiovascular Disease

Studies have consistently shown that humans with a better grip strength have less risk of cancer and cardiovascular disease. A better grip strength is the indicator of strong muscles and bones which is the result of strength training.

7. Strength Training Builds Discipline And Mental Toughness

You build strength by overcoming your body's resistance to step out of its comfort zone. You need the discipline to train consistently. Mental toughness is essentially the ability to push through resistance and be disciplined enough for consistency. The mental toughness you build by strength training transfers to the other areas of your life where you need mental toughness to succeed.

8. Strength Training Decreases Stress And Fights Depression

Strength training is proven to reduce cortisol and increase endorphin release in your brain which leads to less stress and a better feeling of well-being.

9. Strength Training Boosts Self-Esteem And Confidence

Having a lean, strong, healthy, and attractive body will boost your confidence and posture, which will lead to improving your self-esteem.

10. Strength Training Prevents Injury

People tend to refrain from strength training thinking that it's risky but in reality, it's riskier to be weak. They are injured during simple activities such as picking up a book from a shelf or tying their shoes. Almost every friend or relative of mine suffers from a kind of muscle or bone related injury yet they are always worried about me that I will get injured while training for strength. In reality, I have a very low risk of injury thanks to the strength of my bones and muscles.

CHAPTER 2: THE BENEFITS OF BODYWEIGHT TRAINING

You don't have to be great to start, but
you have to start to be great.

- Zig Ziglar

Bodyweight training is an excellent form of strength training which provides all the benefits mentioned in the previous chapter.

In addition to the benefits of strength training, bodyweight training provides the following benefits:

1. Bodyweight Training Gets Results Fast

You don't waste valuable time to learn the correct form of exercises because they are easy to learn and bodyweight training is more forgiving of bad form.

2. Bodyweight Training Builds You Muscle Without Going To The Gym

Bodyweight training can be done in the privacy of your home or any other place that has a few square meters of area. The ability to train at home is priceless, especially if you are living in a city with a lot of traffic. It also works wonders when there's no gym in the vicinity of your home.

I built my six pack abs without stepping foot into a commercial gym. If you are like me and travel a lot, the convenience of bodyweight training is priceless. When you plan to travel, you don't worry about interrupting the consistency of your training schedule. You don't worry about being able to find a good gym.

I did bodyweight training in hotel rooms, parks, stadiums, facile gyms at Airbnb apartments and so on. All you need is a few square meters of area and if your training session involves pull-ups, a pull-up bar.

3. Bodyweight Training Saves You Money

You don't need to pay for a gym membership. You don't need a personal trainer. You don't need to buy treadmills or exercise bikes which are both expensive and provide greatly inferior workouts compared to bodyweight training.

A few days after I started bodyweight training, I bought a pull-up bar and installed it in my house. It cost me around 10 bucks if I am remembering correctly. And that's it. No other costs.

4. Bodyweight Training Saves You Time

Bodyweight training sessions are short yet efficient, energizing and powerful.

Lots of people have trouble finding the time to work out. Not a problem with bodyweight training. As you get better and better (and you will), the workouts take shorter and shorter time. This is because progressive overload at bodyweight training (which you will learn in detail in the progressive overload chapter) is mainly accomplished by completing the same workout in less time.

I can go anywhere in the world and squeeze in a full training session that takes less than 20 minutes.

On the other hand, cardio is extremely time inefficient, ineffective and boring. I shudder when I think about the long hours I wasted on a treadmill at a time when I didn't know any better.

5. Bodyweight Training Is Indiscriminate

You can benefit from bodyweight training regardless of your gender, age, height or present build.

Some men (and most women) don't want to get too big and bulky. They just want that toned, athletic look. Bodyweight training can give you that.

Some people want to get stronger but are intimidated by lifting weights. They can do bodyweight training and get strong.

Some people are beginners. They want to start strength training but don't know where to start. They can start with bodyweight training.

Some people are old. Lifting weights seem impossible to them (which I disagree with by the way). They can do bodyweight training.

Some people are out of shape. These people should not be discouraged that they are not fit enough to do bodyweight training. Every bodyweight exercise included in this book has an easier version which you will see in the exercises chapter. They can start with the easier version until they build the necessary strength to do the full version.

For example, when I started bodyweight training, I was so out of shape that I wasn't able to muster a single pull-up. I did negative pull-ups (the easy version of pull-ups which you will learn in the exercises chapter) until I built the necessary strength to do a regular pull-up.

6. Bodyweight Training Improves Your Endurance And Stamina

Bodyweight training is essentially a high-intensity strength training regimen. High-intensity training improves your endurance and stamina.

7. Bodyweight Training Makes You Look Good Naked

When you build a fit, lean and strong body, you will look terrific naked. Women will go "wow" when you take off your shirt. And of course, sex will be much more enjoyable with women who genuinely and passionately desire you.

CHAPTER 3: MUSCLE BUILDING MINDSET

The worst thing I can be is the same as everybody else.
– Arnold Schwarzenegger

Next time you are out, take a look around. You will see that more than 90% of the people are out of shape. It's easy to see that when you are in shape, you automatically put yourself among the top 10%. When you get muscular, you will be in the top 1% because there are not many people who are both in shape and muscular at the same time.

Why Most People Are Out Of Shape

Everybody wants a lean, strong and athletic body but few people achieve it because of a few reasons:

1. The general public has no idea how to build muscle or burn body fat. I am not blaming them because I was the same too. The conventional wisdom about fitness and diet is false and since the fitness industry is a lucrative one, there are many marketers who push the products that don't work, which confuses people further. Many people believe that building muscle or losing fat are complex issues. They are not.

2. Burning fat is tough and building muscle is tougher. The average man is unable to delay gratification and think long term. He is always on the lookout for shortcuts. Un-

fortunately, there are no shortcuts to success. Any type of success requires a process. People want to skip the process and attain the results by taking shortcuts, which provides a rich soil for scammers to grow. They will burn their money with expensive diet pills or exercise machines which only make their wallets thinner and leaner, not their bodies.

The Importance Of Pushing Through Your Body's Reluctance

Building muscle doesn't happen overnight. The bodyweight training routines you'll find in this book (especially the main routine) are intense. They require mental toughness to start and more mental toughness to complete. There will be times when you will be reluctant to start training. Even when you start training, there will be times when your body will beg you to quit your training prematurely.

It's of utmost importance to complete all the reps in your training session. When the going gets tough and you feel like you can't continue training, don't give up so easily. Wait until you get yourself together, wait for your breathing to catch up, and then resume your training. It doesn't matter how many sets it takes to complete the given number of reps in your routine. Even when you have to rest for 5 minutes just to do 1 more rep, then do it like that. If you are certain that you can't do the proper form of the exercises anymore due to fatigue, switch to the easier version and keep going until you complete all your reps. You should complete all your reps without making excuses. The only exception is when you feel extraordinary pain in a particular body part. Pain is different than fatigue and you will know it when it happens. In case of pain, don't push further. In all the other times, there is no reason to quit your training session prematurely.

The Importance Of Completing Your Workouts

Completing training sessions is of utmost importance because the last few reps of your exercise are the ones that will build you the most muscle. Some bodybuilders are known to ignore the first reps and only count the last few reps because those are the reps that actually count for building muscle.

Everything you do until the last few reps are just a preparation for the real thing. If you will quit your training session prematurely, you might as well not start to train at all. As you progress, you will see that you will get faster and stronger in a very short time provided that you don't quit or cheat.

The Importance Of Honesty

Always be honest with yourself. Honesty is one of the most important things in the muscle game. It sounds unbelievable for someone to not be honest with himself but that's exactly what happens with most people. It's human nature (I guess) to rationalize your shortcomings as unimportant or believe them to not exist at all, but nobody is perfect and everybody has shortcomings. Being honest about your shortcomings will make it possible for you to overcome them.

I can't emphasize being honest about your training enough, because it's common for the human mind to make excuses not to train or to quit training prematurely when the going gets tough.

The "No Excuses" Mindset

I trained when I came back from a long day at work after 10 p.m. and I had to be in bed at 11 p.m. for tomorrow's work day. I trained when it was 90 degrees outside and the air conditioning wasn't working. I trained in hotel rooms when everybody else was out enjoying their vacation. It's easy to find excuses to skip the day's training or to quit training when you feel tired. It's tough to have a no excuses mindset. That's why it's called mental "toughness".

How It Pays To Be Disciplined

Luckily, if you train honestly, you'll see your body changing for good within a few weeks. When you begin to notice your body starting to change, you will be happy, proud and motivated for more. Your friends, family, colleagues, and the women will start telling you that you look great. Your health will improve. Your energy levels will go up. When you push through the initial stages of hardship, you will start reaping the rewards rather quickly. You can then be proud of yourself because you earned it with your honest, hard work. You'll see the first-hand results of discipline. Then you can transfer that attitude to other areas of your life. When the mind believes, the body follows.

CHAPTER 4: EXERCISES

Simplicity is the ultimate sophistication.
-Leonardo da Vinci

The Importance Of Simplicity

I am a huge advocate of simplicity because it gets things done. Simplicity should never fool you as it's hard to believe that most things worth achieving in life are quite simple. Bodybuilding is no exception. You don't need complicated exercises or routines to build a lean, muscular, and athletic body. It's actually the opposite. People who try to do too many things at once get bored quickly and they never achieve anything worthwhile.

I built my physique through simple exercises and simple routines. I eliminated from my routine the exercises that have little to no effect on my physique goals as they consume time and willpower. The exercises and the routines in this book are simple yet effective.

The Importance Of Full Body Training

Many people try to shortcut the muscle building process by training only the muscles that they deem more important than the other muscles. Some of them only train their arms, the remaining muscles be damned. Some others only train their abs with the hope of getting six-pack abs and ignore the rest of their body. This is the wrong attitude to have.

Your body works as a whole unit. The best way to get strong arms or six-pack abs or any other strong muscle is to train your whole body. The workouts you'll find in this book are designed to train your whole body. No muscle in the body is more important than the other. You must train them all to have a well-built body.

When you do the workouts in this book, you will not only discover your strengths but also you will be able to pinpoint your weaknesses. For example, when I first started strength training, I wasn't able to do a single pull-up. That was frustrating at the time but I started with doing the easy version of pull-ups (negative pull-ups) until I could do a regular pull-up and I quickly built on top of that. Now I can do 30 strict pull-ups in a row.

Don't be surprised if you discover some of your muscles to be weaker than the others. I will give you the easier versions of each exercise so that you can still train without missing your sessions. I never skipped a training session that includes pull-ups just because I couldn't do a proper pull-up since I could replace the regular pull-ups with negative pull-ups which are easier to do.

After you work out for a while, you will have a clear understanding of your body so that you can design your workout schedule targeting your weaknesses. Just stick with the 12-week routine(s) in this book until you discover your strengths and weaknesses. Then you can design your own training routine to work more on your weaknesses and less on your strengths. It's entirely possible that any weakness you currently have may well be cured by the time you finish your program.

The 8 Best Bodyweight Exercises

There are only 8 exercises that you will be doing over and over again during your program. These exercises are simple yet extremely powerful. They are all compound exercises where you work more than one muscle group at the same time, which will give you the most bang for your buck.

Here are the 8 exercises and the muscles they work:

- **Burpee** (abs, triceps, obliques, shoulders, chest, quads, glutes, hamstrings, calves, the adonis belt)
- **Pull-up** (back, shoulders, biceps, forearms)
- **Push-up** (chest, shoulders, triceps, abs, anterior)
- **Sit-up** (abs, obliques, tensors, thighs)
- **Squat** (hamstrings, quadriceps, glutes, adductors, calves, abs)
- **Leg raise** (abs, thighs, obliques)
- **Lunge** (quadriceps, hamstrings, glutes, calves, abs, back)
- **Jump** (quadriceps, hip flexors, hamstrings, calves)

All the exercises will also work your cardiovascular system as the workouts are high-intensity. The more muscles you employ with a specific exercise, the more your cardiovascular system will work. Burpees are the best in that regard since the burpee is the exercise that trains the most muscle groups at the same time. This is also one of the reasons why you have multiple exercises for a group of muscle. The more you employ your cardiovascular system, the quicker you will get exhausted, so it's best to superset the exercises to avoid burnouts before you get the most out of your workout.

Performing The Exercises

It's best to perform all the exercises in full, proper form. But, there will probably be times where you are unable to perform the full version of a particular exercise.

When I started bodyweight training, I was unable to do a proper pull-up so I started by doing the easier version (negative pull-ups). As I grew stronger, I was finally able to start doing proper pull-ups for a few reps, then I would proceed with the remaining reps by switching to negative pull-ups again. It took me a while to perform all the pull-ups in proper form during a particular training session. Don't get discouraged when you discover that you can't perform a particular exercise in proper form. Proceed with the easier version until you build up enough strength to perform the full version.

Not being able to perform the full version of any exercise can happen at the beginning of a training session or when you are well into the session. For example, if you are unable to do a push-up even when you are fresh and rested, you start with the easy version. As you keep on doing the easy version for a while, you will build up enough strength to muster up a full one. If you start by doing the full version but you can no longer do it, switch to the easier version.

For example, you can start your session by doing full, proper push-ups but you may find yourself no longer able to do another full push-up. If this happens, it's not an excuse to quit your training session before you complete all the reps. Keep on training by doing the easy version of push-ups until you complete all the reps in your session. Same goes for other exercises. If you can't even do the easy version, wait for a few minutes (or as many minutes as it takes) until your muscles recover and proceed with your training. There's no excuse (other than injury) to quit your training until you complete all the reps (full or easy version) in your workout, no matter how long it takes.

Burpee

The burpee is the king of all bodyweight exercises because it works the largest groups of your muscles at once. With each rep of burpees, you train your abs, triceps, obliques, shoulders, chest, quads, glutes, hamstrings, calves and the adonis belt.

Burpees also boost your cardiovascular capacity because when you work the most of your muscles in your body at once, they will need oxygen. You will notice that you will start to breathe heavily after a few reps of burpees. That's completely normal so don't freak out.

Burpees not only build your muscles and boost your cardiovascular capacity but also improve your mental strength. No matter how well-trained you are, burpees will become difficult to do after a few reps. You will have to employ your mental powers to keep on doing burpees until you reach your target rep count.

This mental and physical effort will not be in vain though, because you will notice that after a few weeks of doing burpees regularly, your muscles will improve noticeably and you will feel a lot more athletic compared to just a few weeks before. Burpees are extremely rewarding in this regard and the benefits don't end there. Burpees burn calories which will make it easier to shed pounds of fat off your body.

How To Do A Burpee With The Proper Form

A proper burpee is the one with the push-up movement included.

1. Start with a standing position with your feet shoulder-width apart.
2. Squat and place your hands in front of you on the floor.
3. Shoot your feet back and get into a push-up position.
4. Do a push-up. Your chest briefly touches the ground.
5. Push your feet back to their original position.
6. Jump into the air and clap your arms over your head.
7. Repeat.

BURPEE PROPER FORM IN PICTURES

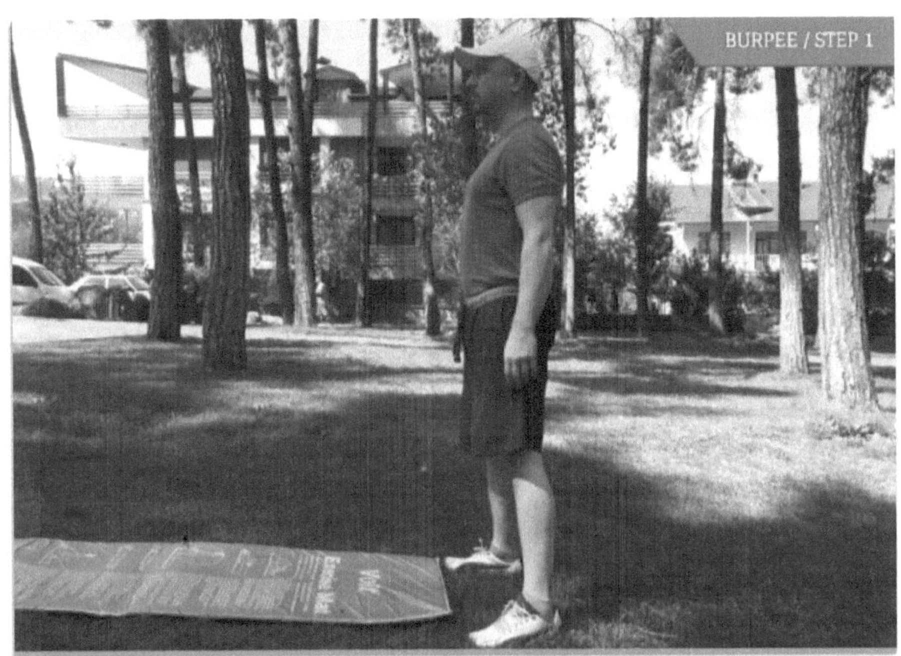
BURPEE / STEP 1

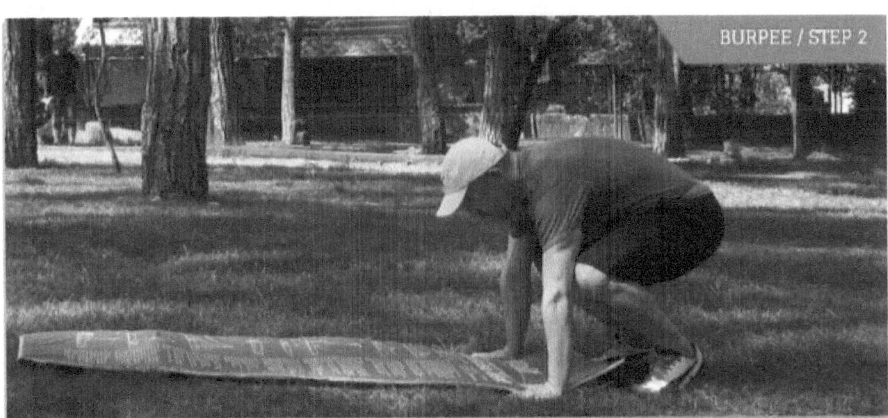
BURPEE / STEP 2

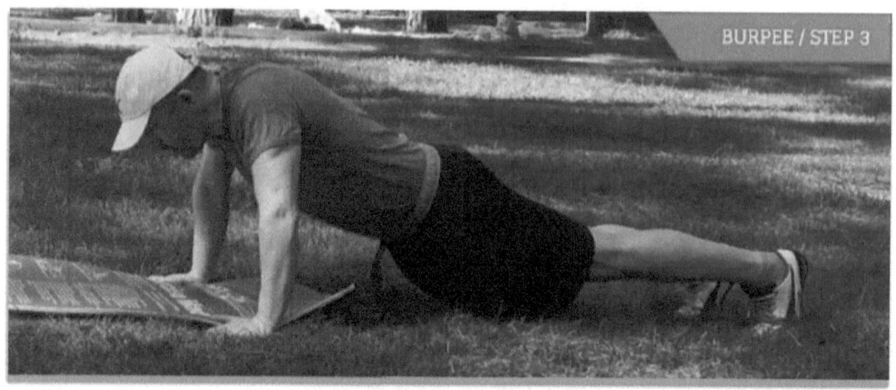
BURPEE / STEP 3

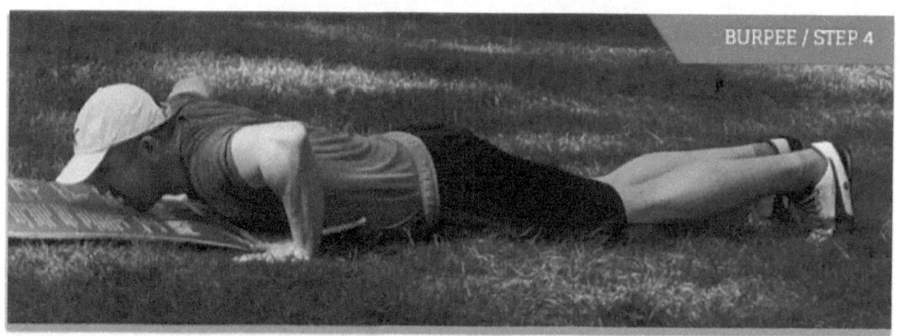
BURPEE / STEP 4

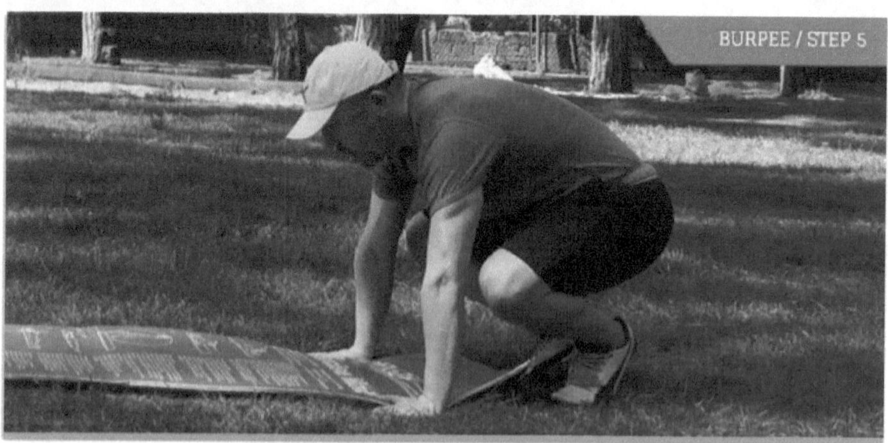
BURPEE / STEP 5

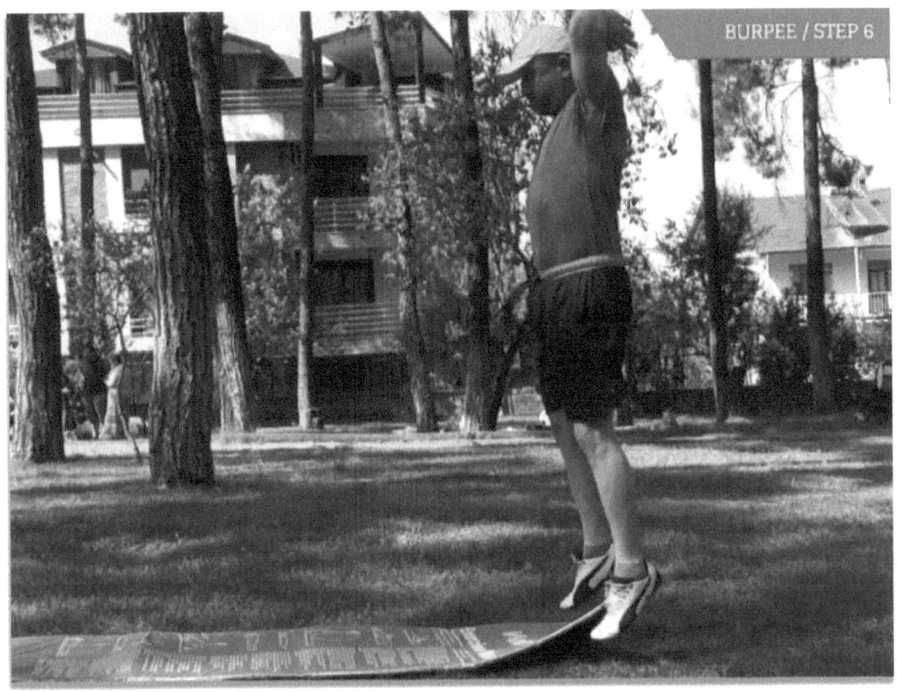

The Easy Version Of The Burpee (Modified Burpee)

The easy version of the burpee is the one without the push-up movement.

1. Start with a standing position with your feet shoulder-width apart.
2. Squat and place your hands in front of you on the floor.
3. Shoot your feet back and get into a push-up position.
4. Push your feet back to their original position.
5. Jump into the air and clap your arms over your head.
6. Repeat.

MODIFIED BURPEE IN PICTURES

Modified burpee is the proper burpee without the push-up part. Refer to the proper burpee pictures above and skip the step 4.

Pull-Up

The pull-up is one of the most challenging but also one of the most rewarding muscle building exercises.

A person who can do a proper pull-up is considered to be fit. Most people can't do a single proper pull-up if their lives depended on it.

If you can't do a proper pull-up, don't fret. You will get there if you follow the guidelines in this book.

When you look around the internet or watch other people train, you will notice that the pull-up has various versions. Some people do it with an overhand grip, others do it with an underhand grip (chin-ups), and a few others do it with a neutral grip. Some people do it with a wide grip (thinking that it will build them a wider back), and others do it with a close grip.

To understand which combination of the grip styles produce the best results, we must understand the purpose of pull-ups.

Pull-ups are meant to target your back muscles. Doing pull-ups is a great way to build a big, muscular, and wide back. Pull-ups work your arms and shoulders too but the main point of doing pull-ups is to train your back. There's nothing wrong with training your shoulders and arms but there are other exercises to train them better. When you do pull-ups, your aim is to develop your back muscles.

The problem with gripping the bar overhand, underhand or wide is that you put too much pressure on your arms and shoulders. For example, when you perform a chin-up (the one with the underhand grip), you will put too much pressure on your biceps, which is a small muscle group. After a few reps, your biceps will start to fatigue and you will have to quit before your back muscles are properly trained. Doing pull-ups with an overhand grip is better but your arm muscles will still get fatigued before your back muscles.

There is a similar problem with wide-grip pull-ups. When you grip the bar wide while doing pull-ups, your arms are doing most of the work. Again, your arm muscles will give up before you properly work your back muscles.

The best grip for pull-ups is the grip that puts the least strain on your arms. That grip is the neutral, close grip.

So, whenever your training session requires you to do pull-ups, it means that you are better off if you perform neutral, close grip pull-ups. That's the best type of grip to build a bigger and wider back. Don't skip the pull-ups though if your pull-up bar doesn't allow you to grip the bar neutrally. In that case, do overhand, close grip pull-ups.

How To Do A Pull-Up With The Proper Form

1. Start with a standing position.
2. Grab the bar and grip it (preferably neutral with a narrow grip, if not, overhand with shoulder-width grip).
3. Get your feet off the floor and lock your arms out.
4. Pull yourself up and get your chin above the bar.
5. Get back down to your initial gripping position.
6. Repeat from step 2.

PULL-UP PROPER FORM IN PICTURES

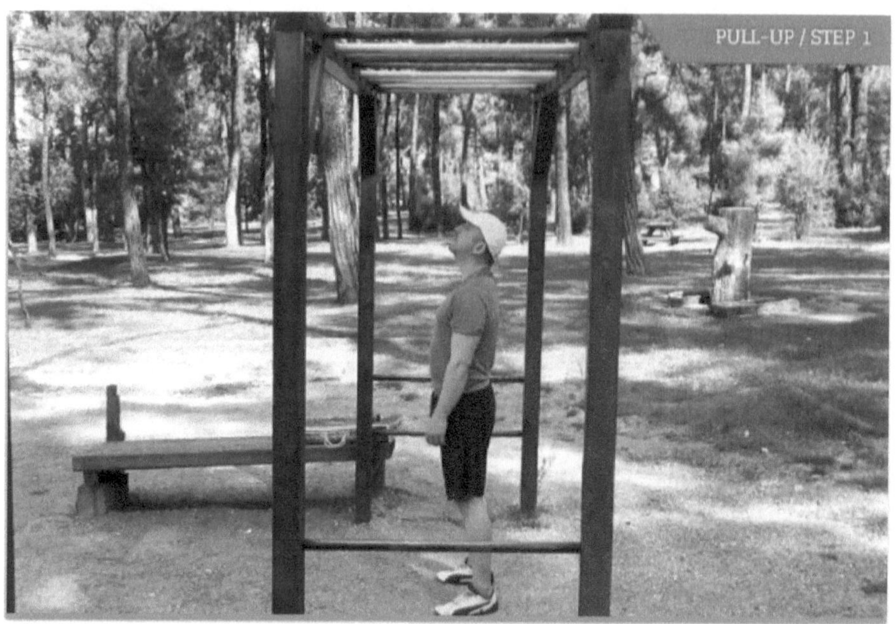
PULL-UP / STEP 1

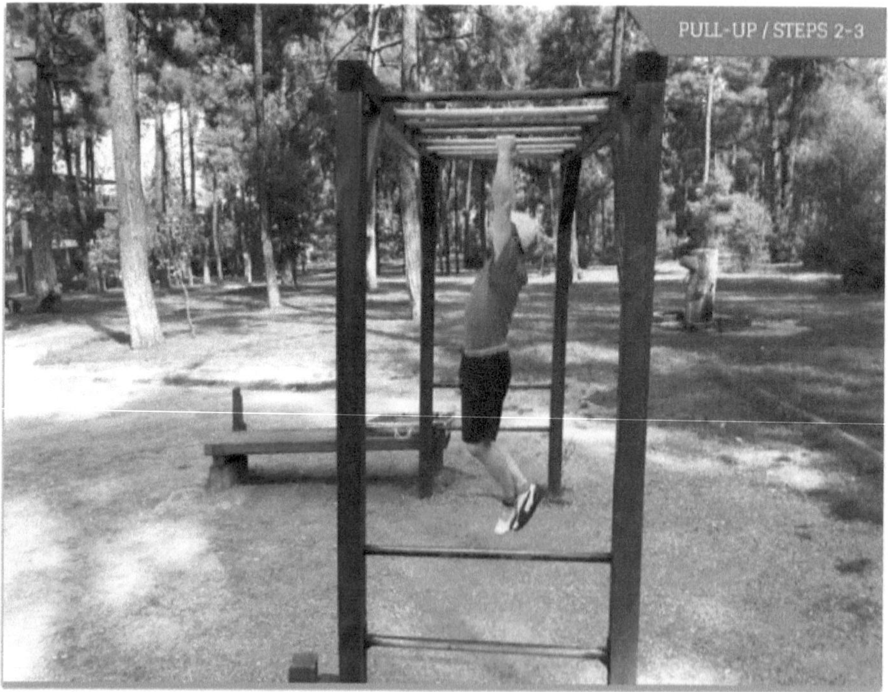
PULL-UP / STEPS 2-3

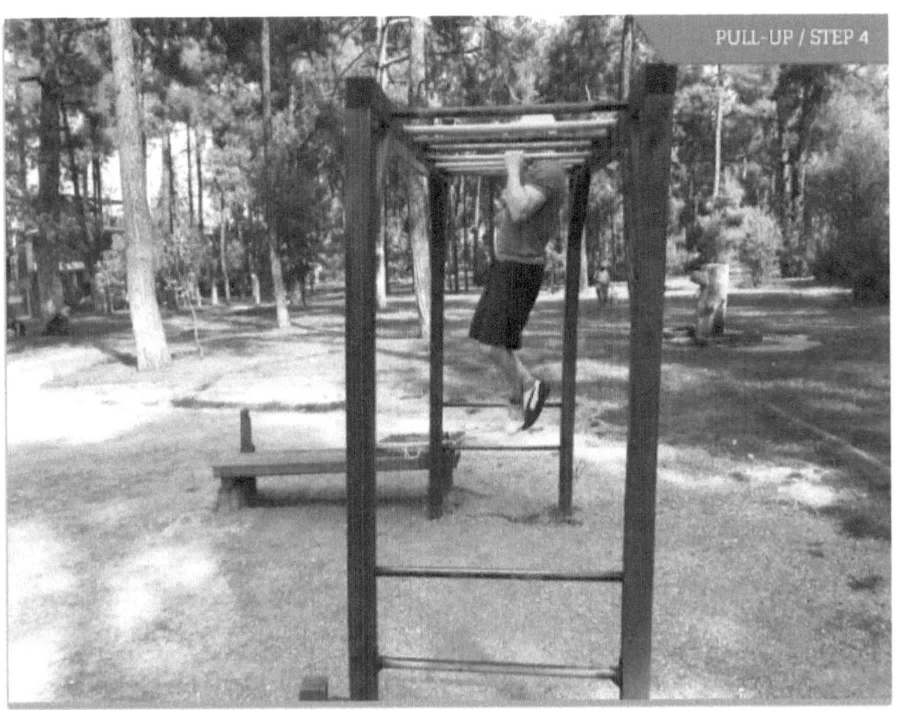
PULL-UP / STEP 4

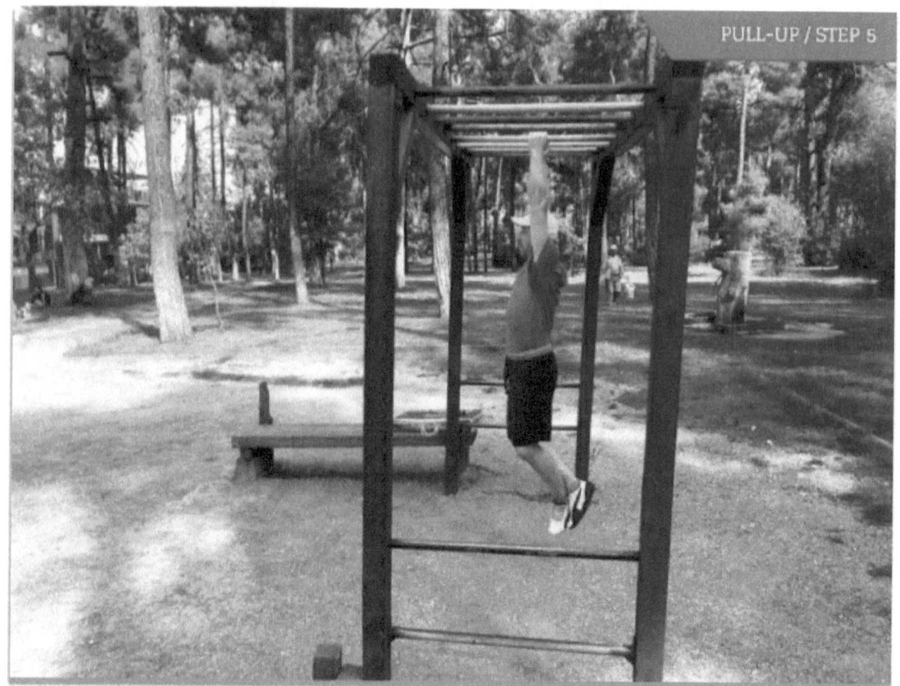

Repeat from step 2.

The Easy Version Of The Pull-Up (Negative Pull-Up)

The difficult part of the pull-up is the part where you pull yourself up. If you can't pull yourself up (yet), don't be frustrated. Skip the pulling yourself up part of the pull-up and concentrate on the part where you are lowering yourself down.

1. Grab the bar with your feet on the floor and grip it (preferably neutral with a narrow grip, if not, overhand with shoulder-width grip).
2. Jump up to get your chin above the bar.
3. Lower yourself slowly and in control until you get back down to your initial gripping position.
7. Repeat from step 2.

Doing negative pull-ups is a great way to strengthen your back muscles. When you build up enough strength by doing negative-pullups for a while, you will be able to do a regular pull-up.

Another thing you can do to improve your pull-ups is to lose fat. If you have extra pounds of fat in your body, it will be harder for you to pull yourself up as you will have to lift more weight. When you slim down, you increase your chances to do a proper pull-up, and later increase the number of pull-ups you can do.

NEGATIVE PULL-UP IN PICTURES

You can refer to the pictures of the proper pull-up for the negative pull-up form. While doing negative pull-ups you don't pull yourself up but jump from the ground until your chin is above the bar and you lower yourself slowly and in control until you get back down to your initial gripping position. This motion counts as one rep.

Push-Up

The push-up is another great bodyweight exercise which mainly targets your chest muscles. Since it's a compound exercise, you will train your arms and shoulders as well.

There are many versions of push-ups to target different groups of muscles but you will only do the good-old regular push-ups for the sake of simplicity and efficiency.

Performing a proper push-up is easier than performing burpees or pull-ups but they still can be challenging. If you can't do a regular push-up, there's no shame in performing the easier version until you build enough strength to do them with the proper form.

How To Do A Push-Up With The Proper Form

1. Start with the prone position where you lie flat with

your chest down, back up. Your feet should be shoulder width apart and your hands should be placed wider than shoulder-width apart, touching the ground.
2. Push yourself up and rise on the tip of your feet while your chest, hips, and legs leave the ground.
3. Go up until your arms are straight.
4. Go back down to your starting position.
5. Repeat.

PUSH-UP PROPER FORM IN PICTURES

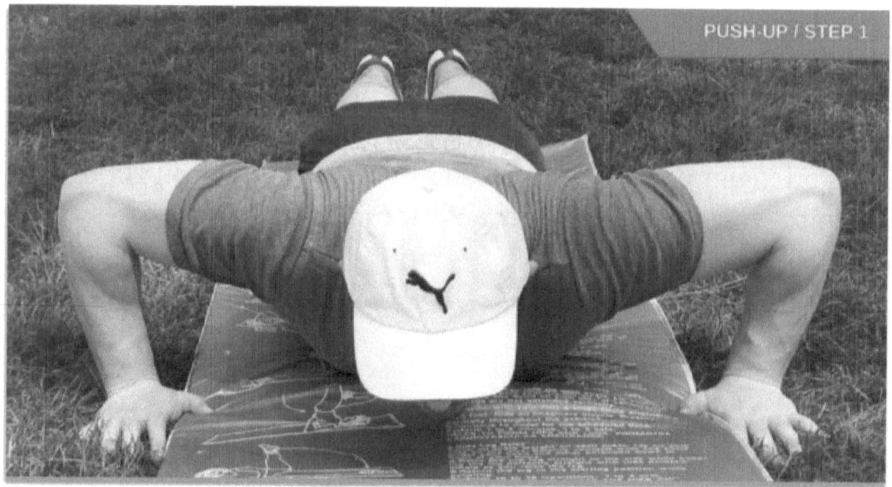

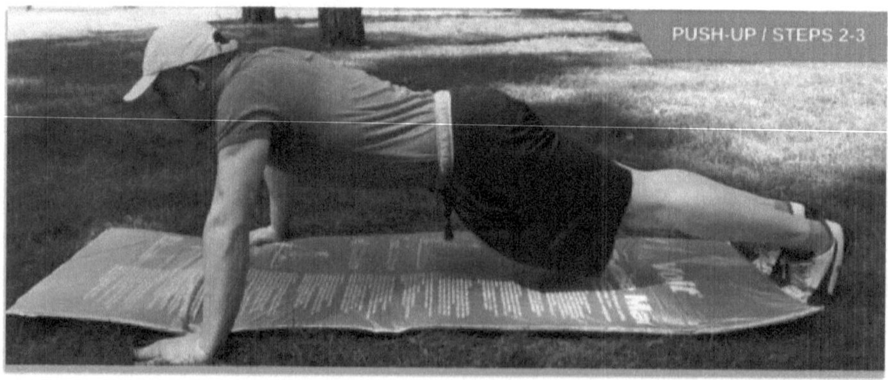

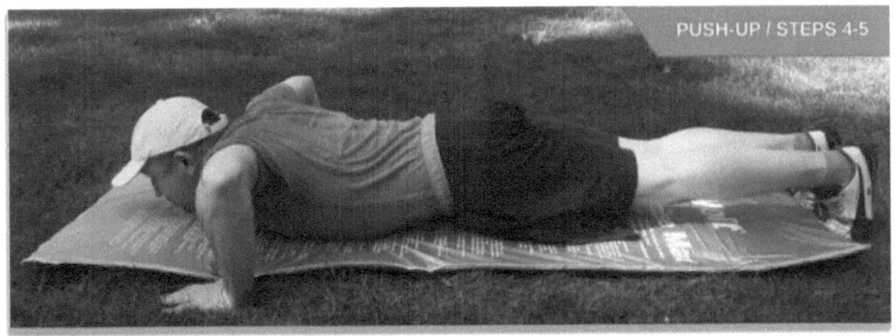

The Easy Version Of The Push-Up (Modified Push-Up)

1. Start with the prone position where you lie flat with your chest down, back up. Your feet should be shoulder width apart and your hands should be placed slightly wider than shoulder-width apart, touching the ground.
2. Push yourself up and rise on your knees while your chest and hips and leave the ground.
3. Go up until your arms are straight.
4. Go back down to your starting position.
5. Repeat.

Doing modified push-ups is a great way to strengthen your chest muscles. When you build up enough strength by doing modified push-ups for a while, you will be able to do a regular push-up. Other exercises will also strengthen your core which will help you with your push-ups. Just like pull-ups, it's always a good idea to lose the extra pounds of fat in your body to increase the number of regular pull-ups you do.

MODIFIED PUSH-UP IN PICTURES

Starting position for the modified push-up is the same as the regular push-up.

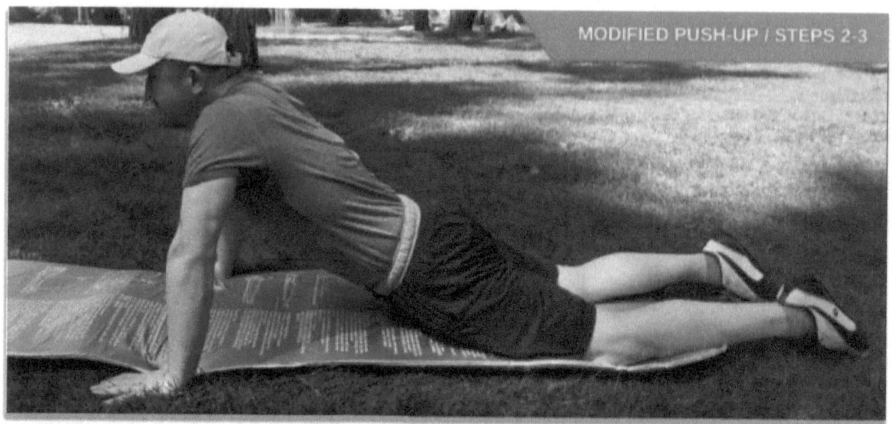

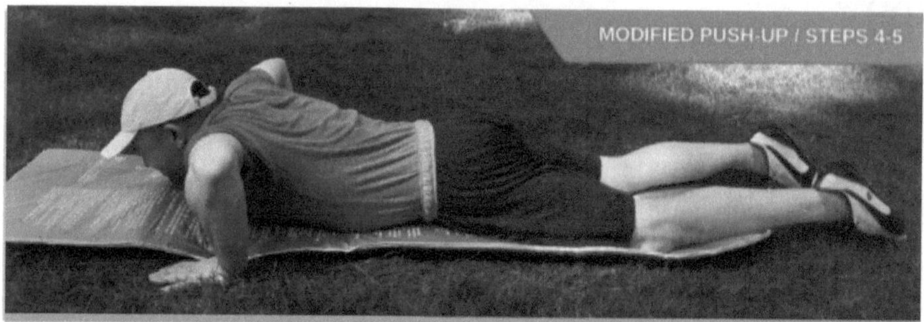

Sit-Up

The sit-up is one of the most commonly performed bodyweight exercises which mainly works your ab muscles. It's a great exercise to strengthen your core, which will help you to perform any other strength training exercise better.

While sit-ups are too popular, many people do them wrong. Here's how to perform a proper sit-up:

How To Do A Sit-Up With The Proper Form

1. Start with a sitting position where your glutes and feet are touching the ground and your feet touching each other. Your hands touch the ground in front of your feet.
2. Swing with arms while you move your body back until

your hands touch the ground behind your head and your back touches the ground.

3. Sit-up with a forward motion with your hands swinging forward until you touch back to the ground in front of your feet.
4. Repeat from step 2.

While sit-ups aren't as challenging as the burpees, pull-ups or push-ups, you can still have trouble performing them properly, especially when the fatigue kicks in during your training sessions. When you find yourself in such a situation, switch to the easy version of sit-ups.

SIT-UP PROPER FORM IN PICTURES

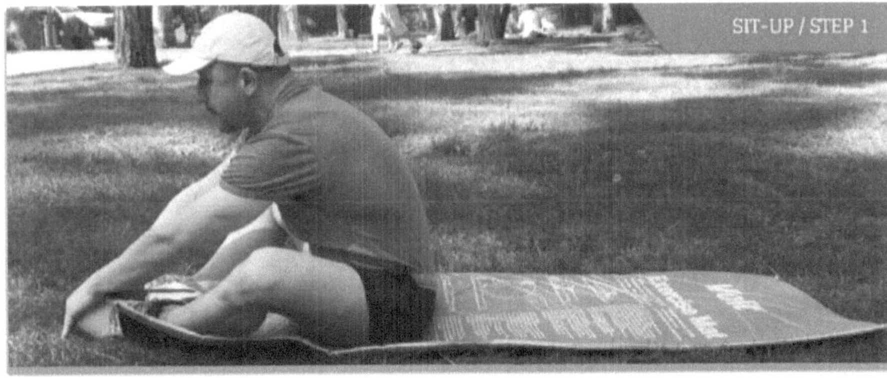

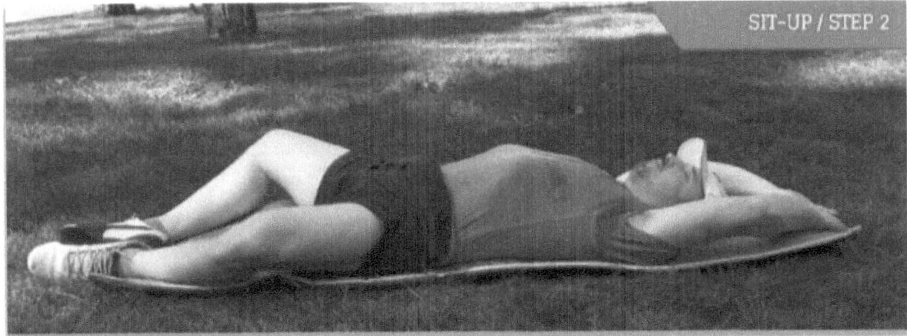

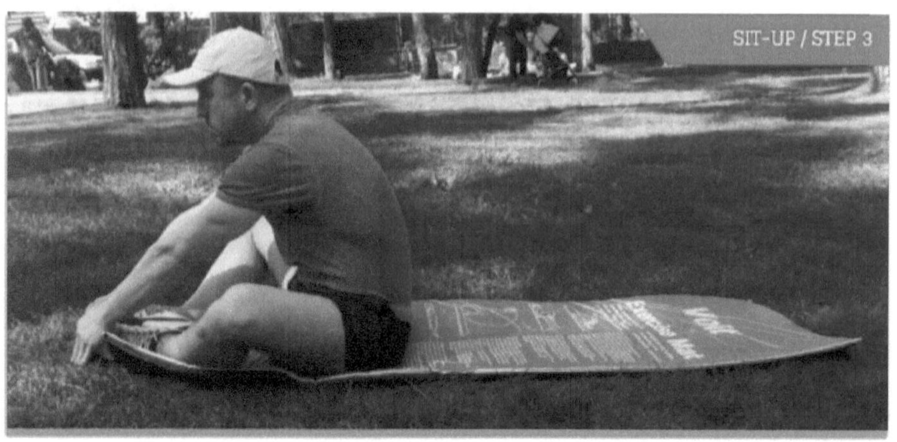

The Easy Version Of The Sit-Up (Modified Sit-Up)

1. Start with a sitting position where your glutes and feet are touching the ground and your feet touching each other. Your hands touch the ground in front of your feet.
2. Swing with arms while you move your body back until your hands touch the ground behind your head and your back touches the ground.
3. Sit-up with a forward motion with your hands swinging forward until you touch your knees with the tip of your hands.
4. Repeat from step 2.

MODIFIED SIT-UP IN PICTURES

Steps 1 and 2 are the same as the proper sit-up. On step 3, you only sit-up until your hands reach your knees.

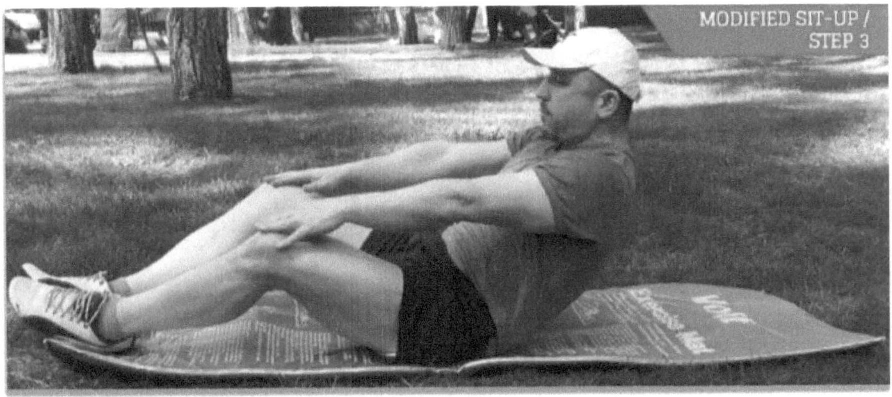

Squat

The bodyweight squat is a great exercise to train your legs. Since it's a compound movement you also get to train your glutes, adductors, and abs.

How To Do A Squat With The Proper Form

1. Start with a standing position with your heels shoulder-width apart. Your feet should be pointing slightly outwards. Your shoulders, hips, knees, and heels must be in a line.
2. Start squatting down by pushing your knees out and keeping your lower back tight. Your knees must NOT bend inwards. They should be bending outwards. Your shoulders and heels must always be in a line during the whole of the movement. Give your weight to your heels.
3. Squat down until your hips are at least parallel to the ground. Go slightly deeper below your knees if you have the flexibility but parallel is ok.
4. Stand up to return to your starting position.
5. Repeat.

When you find yourself in a position that you can't perform a proper squat due to fatigue or lack of flexibility, proceed with your training by doing the easy version.

SQUAT PROPER FORM IN PICTURES

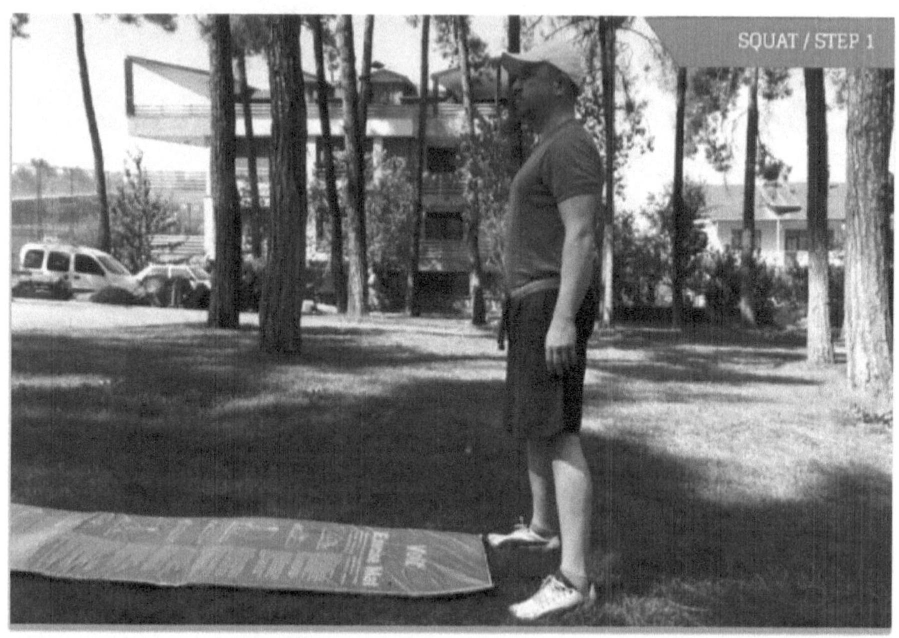

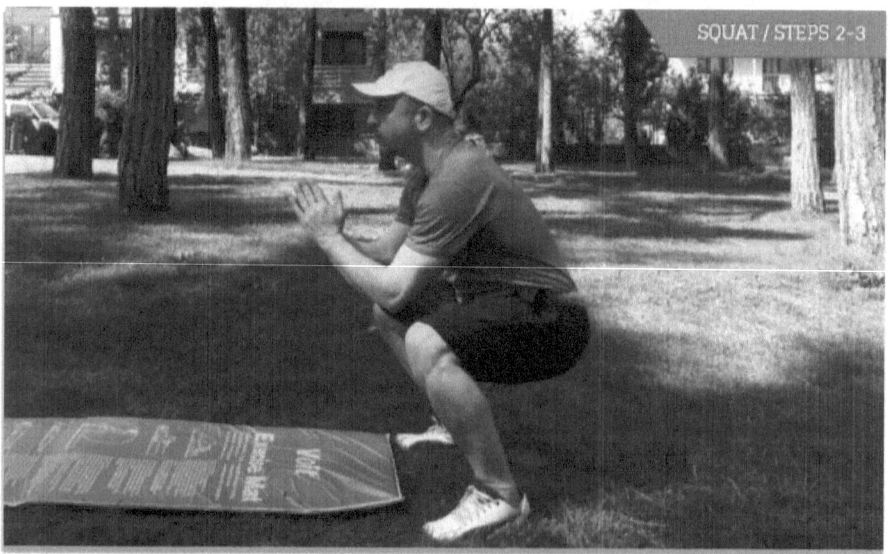

Stand up to your starting position and repeat.

The Easy Version Of The Squat (Modified Squat)

1. Start with a standing position with your heels shoulder-width apart. Your feet should be pointing slightly outwards. Your shoulders, hips, knees, and heels must be in a line
2. Start squatting down by pushing your knees out and keeping your lower back tight. Your knees must NOT bend inwards. They should be bending outwards. Your shoulders and heels must always be in a line throughout the movement. Give your weight to your heels.
3. Squat down as deep as you can go.
4. Stand up to return to your starting position.
5. Repeat.

MODIFIED SQUAT IN PICTURES

Modified squat step 3 is different from regular squat, other steps are the same.

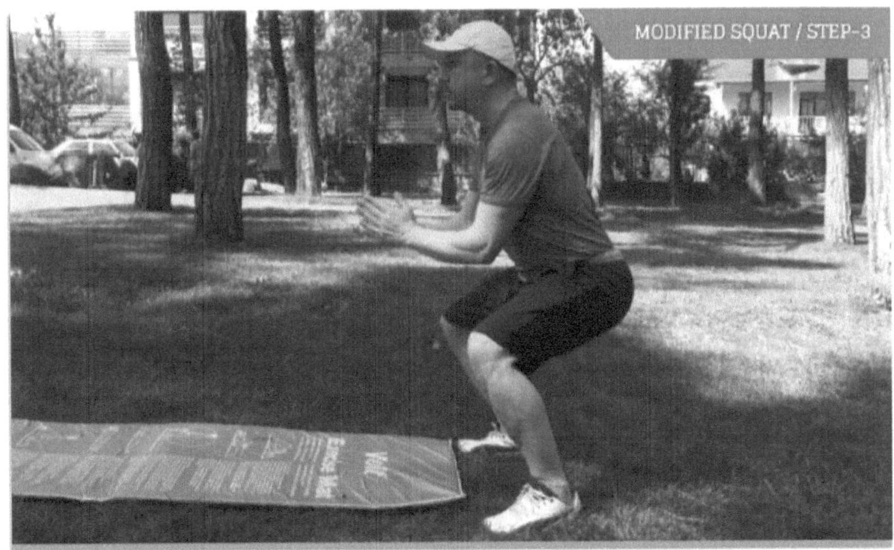

Leg Raise

Leg raise is a great exercise to work your abs (especially the lower parts of your abdomens) and the stabilizing muscles around your core. It also works your thighs and obliques.

How To Do A Leg Raise With The Proper Form

1. Start with the supine position where you lie flat with your back down, chest up. Place your hands lying flat on the ground next to your body. Your feet should contact and your legs should be straight at all times.
2. Press your lower back on the ground and lift your legs up until they are vertical to the ground.
3. Get your legs and feet back to the starting position.
4. Repeat from step 2.

After doing a certain number of reps with leg raises or when your legs lack the flexibility to raise your legs up until they are vertical to the ground, you can do the easy version of the leg raises.

LEG RAISE PROPER FORM IN PICTURES

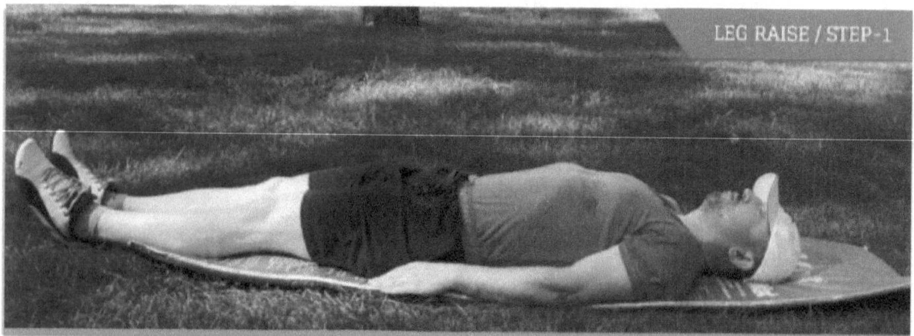

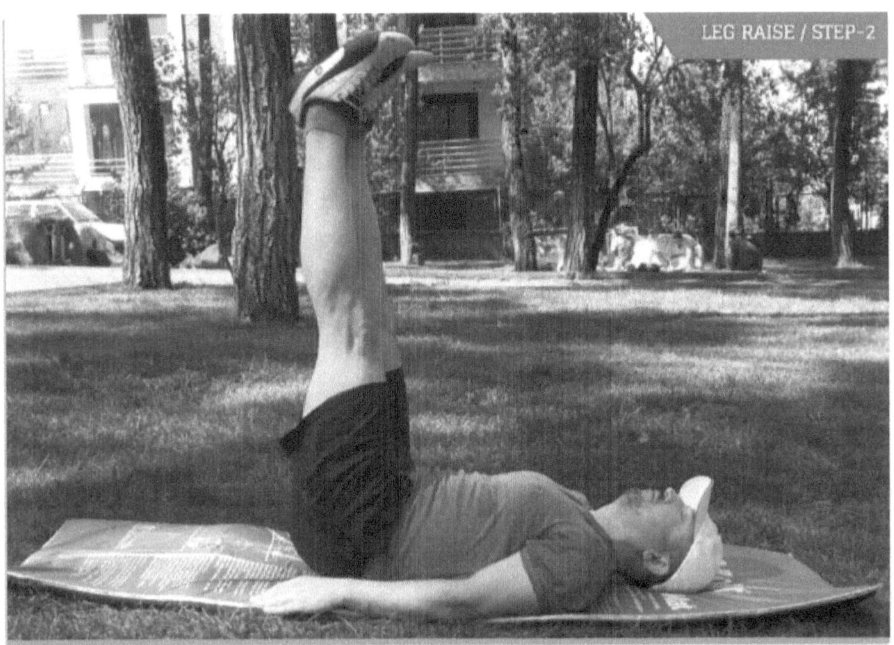

Get your legs and feet back to the position at step 1 and repeat.

The Easy Version Of The Leg Raise (Modified Leg Raise)

1. Start with the supine position where you lie flat with your back down, chest up. Place your hands lying flat on the ground next to your body. Your feet should contact and your legs should be straight at all times.
2. Press your lower back on the ground and lift your legs up as high as you can.
3. Get your legs and feet back to the starting position.
4. Repeat from step 2.

MODIFIED LEG RAISE IN PICTURES

Only step-2 of the modified leg raise is different from the proper leg raise:

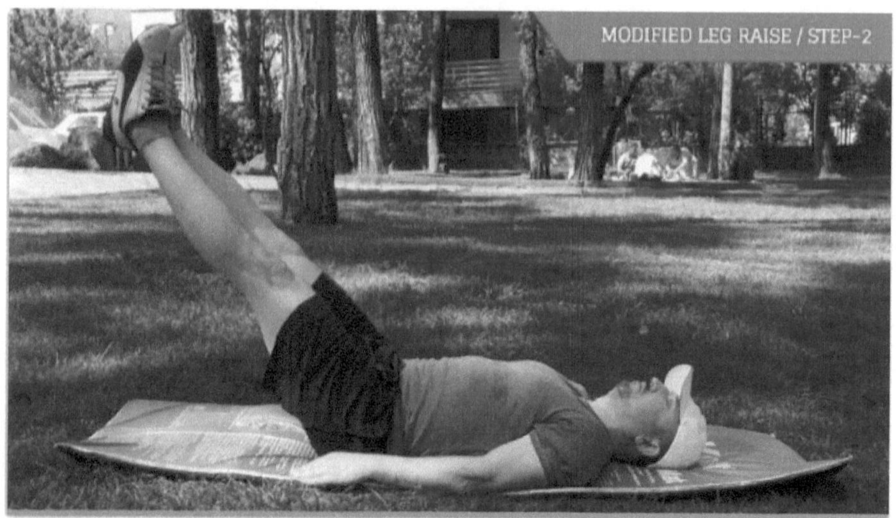

Lunge

The lunge is a great exercise to train your quadriceps muscles and the stabilizer muscles around them. They also work your hamstrings, glutes, calves, abs, and back.

How To Do A Lunge With The Proper Form

1. Start with a standing position with your feet shoulder-width apart and your palms resting over your hips. Your shoulders, hips, knees, and heels should be in a line. Your hands should be on your hips during the whole movement.
2. Lunge forward with one of your legs until your knee touches the ground while keeping your back and thigh vertical to the ground.
3. Get back up to the starting position.
4. Lunge forward with your other leg until your knee touches the ground while keeping your back and thigh vertical to the ground.
5. Get back up to the starting position.
6. Repeat with the other leg and vice versa.

Each leg counts as a rep.

If your quadriceps or stabilizer muscles aren't strong enough (yet) or you get fatigued during your workout that you can't do the lunges with the proper form, you can proceed with your training by doing the easier version.

LUNGE PROPER FORM IN PICTURES

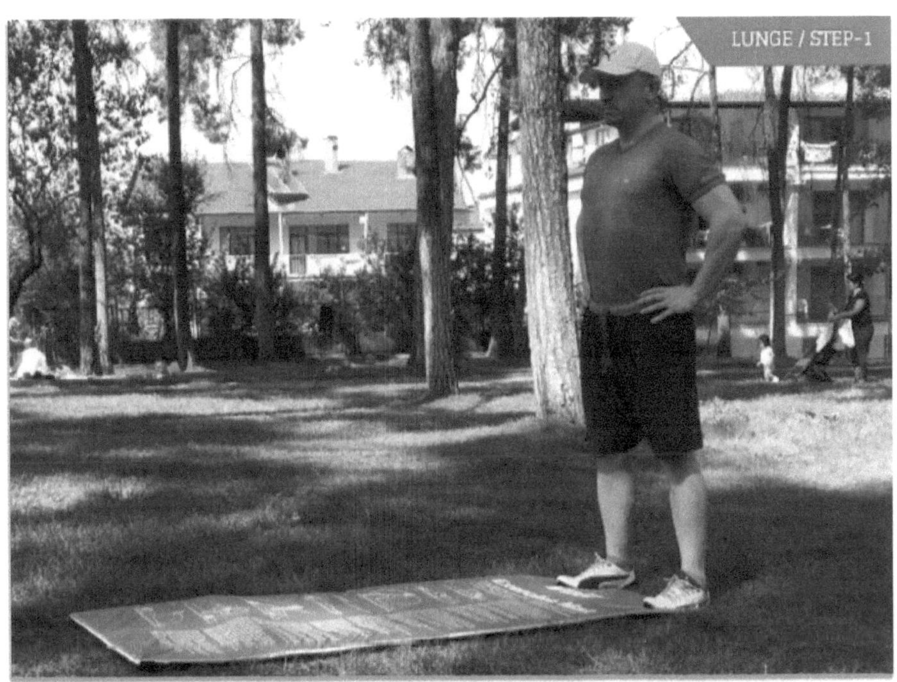

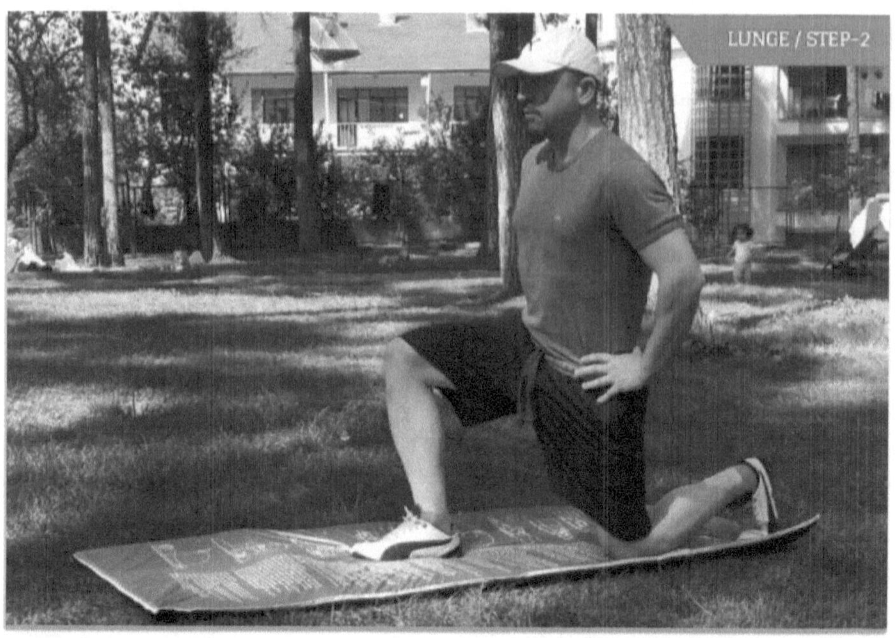
LUNGE / STEP-2

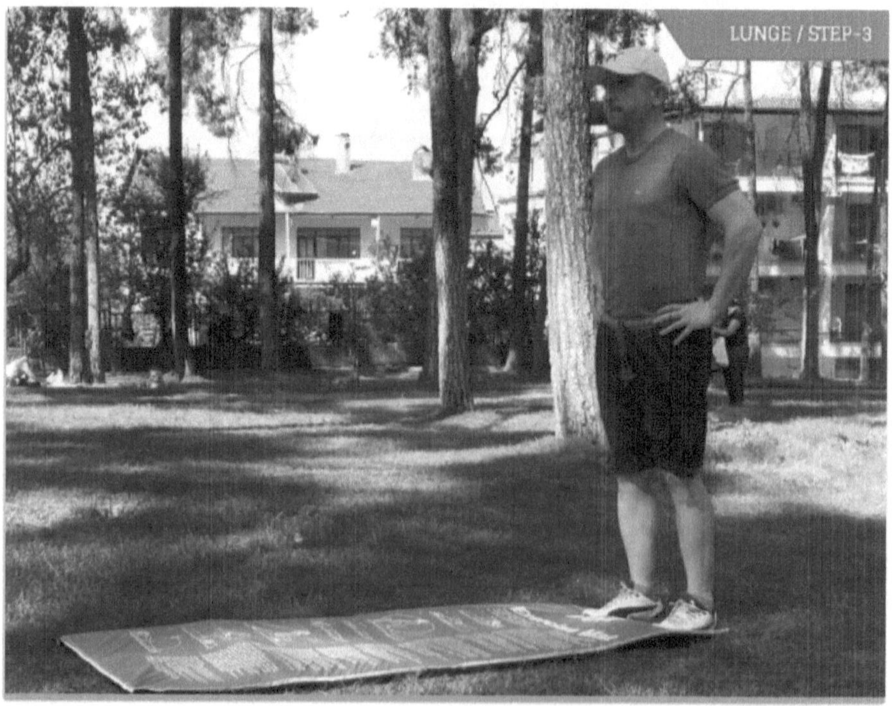
LUNGE / STEP-3

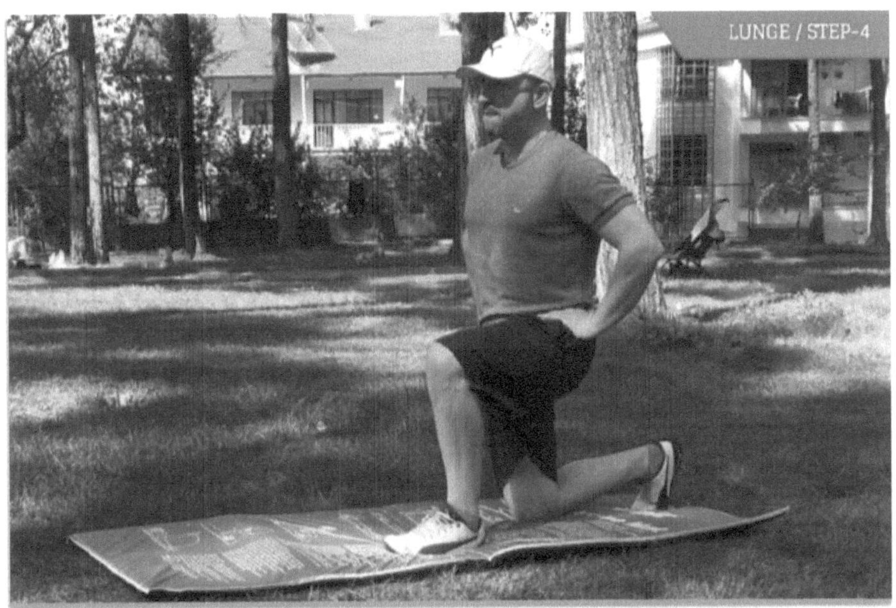

Get back to the starting position and repeat with the other leg as pictured in steps 1 and 2.

The Easy Version Of The Lunge (Modified Lunge)

1. Start with a standing position with your feet shoulder-width apart and your palms resting over your hips. Your shoulders, hips, knees, and heels should be in a line.
2. Lunge forward with one of your legs until your knee touches the ground while keeping your back and thigh vertical to the ground.
3. Get back up to the starting position with the help of your hand supporting your leg.
4. Lunge forward with your other leg until your knee touches the ground while keeping your back and thigh vertical to the ground.
5. Get back up to the starting position with the help of your hand supporting your leg.
6. Repeat with the other leg and vice versa.

Each leg counts as a rep.

MODIFIED LUNGE IN PICTURES

During modified lunges, you use your hands to help you with the movement when you are lunging forward and getting back up. Starting position is the same.

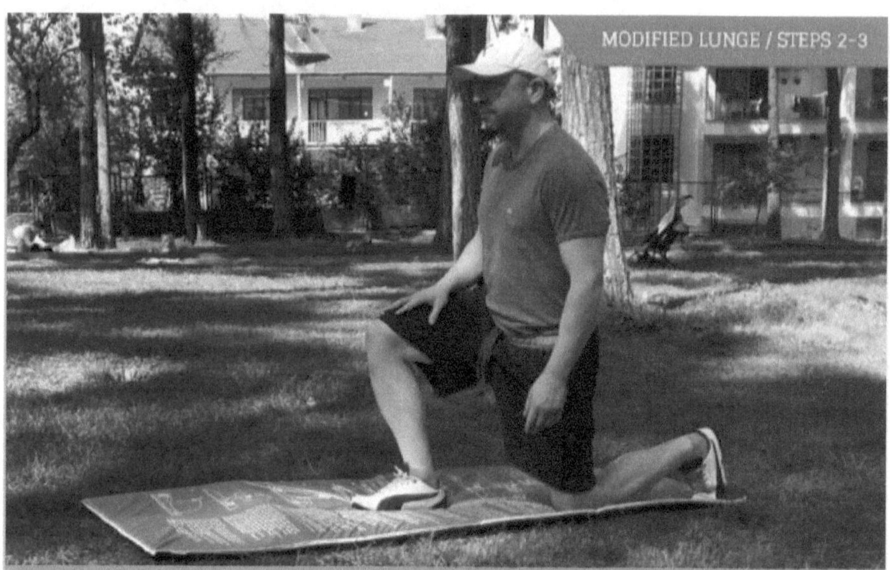

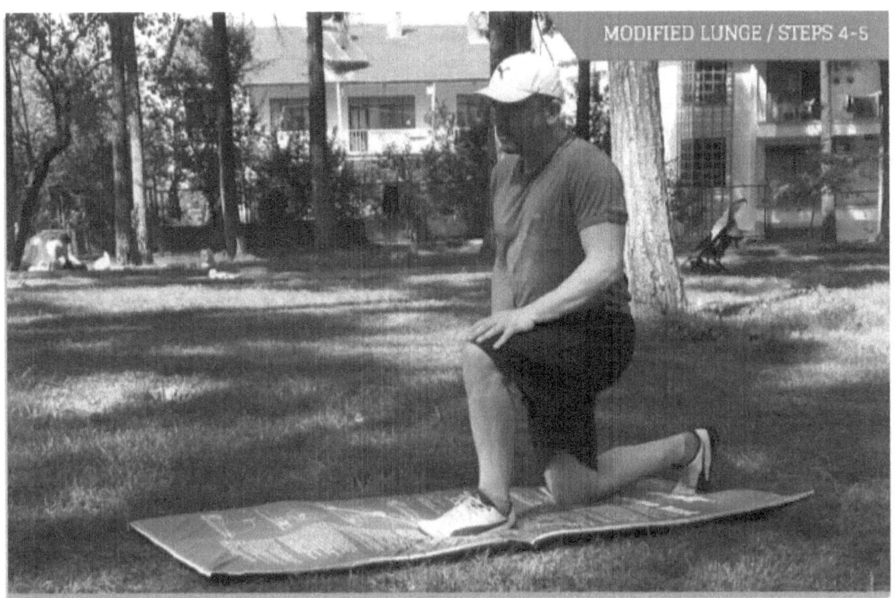

Jump

Jump is a great exercise to work your legs and cardiovascular system. It's also a great way to train your hip flexors.

How To Do A Jump With The Proper Form

1. Start with a standing position with your feet shoulder-width apart
2. Jump with both feet at the same time
3. Raise your knees up until the hip level or higher. Be careful not to turn your knees in.
4. Land on your feet to get back to the starting position.
5. Repeat.

If you find yourself too fatigued to jump up to the hip level or you lack the flexibility, proceed with the easier version.

JUMP PROPER FORM IN PICTURES

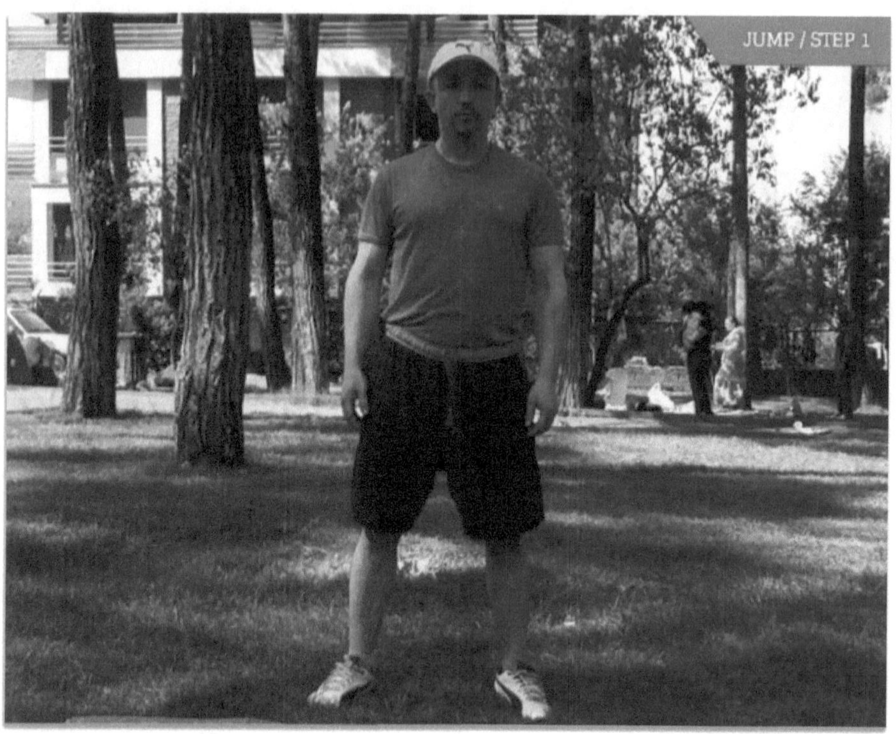
JUMP / STEP 1

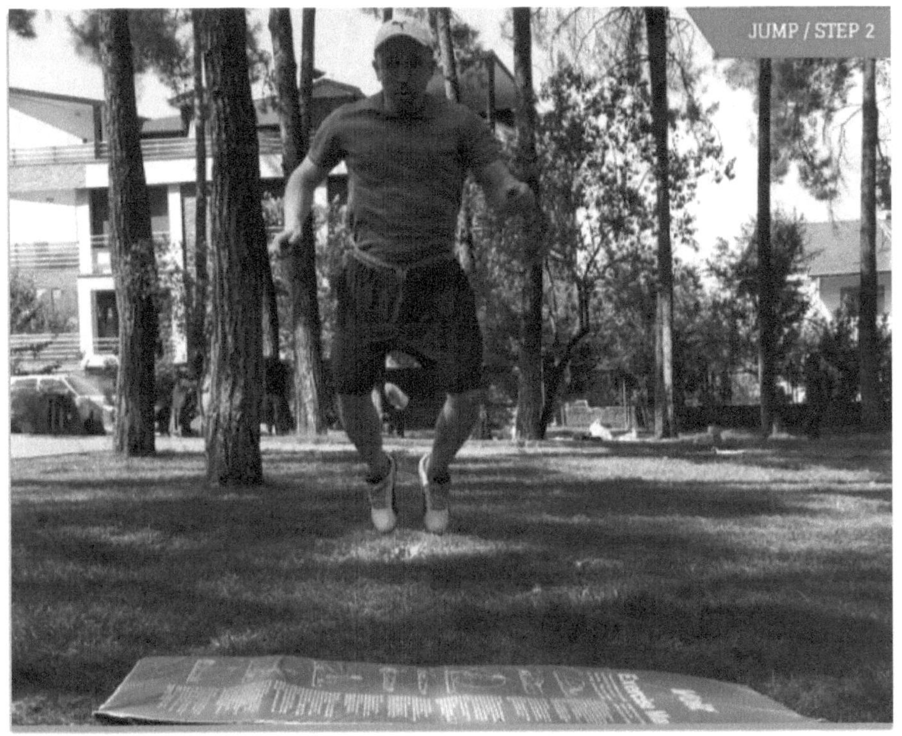
JUMP / STEP 2

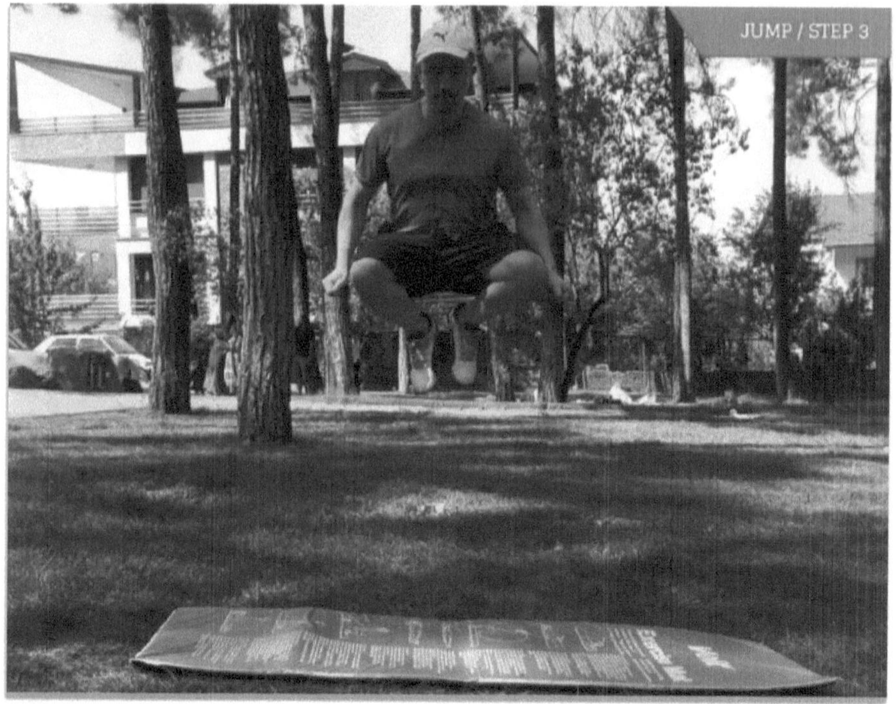

Land on your feet and repeat.

The Easy Version Of The Jump (Modified Jump)

1. Start with a standing position with your feet shoulder-width apart
2. Jump with both feet at the same time
3. Raise your knees up until you can't raise them any longer. Be careful not to turn your knees in.
4. Land on your feet to get back to the starting position.
5. Repeat

MODIFIED JUMP IN PICTURES

Modified jump is different from the proper jump only at step 3.

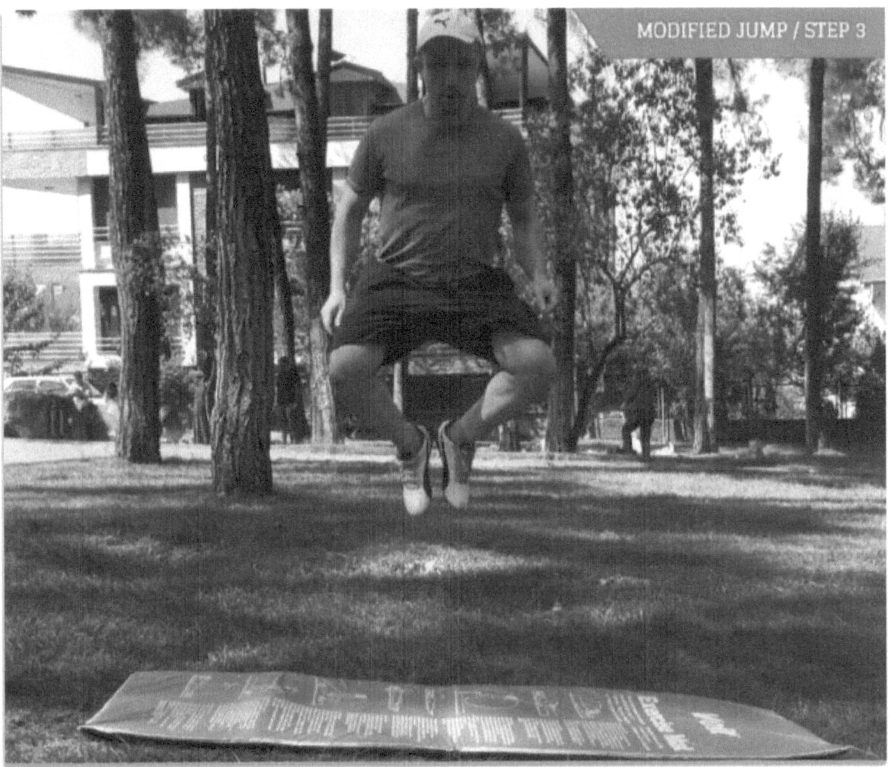

Conclusion

To build a great physique, these 8 exercises are all the exercises you need. Don't be fooled by the fact that the exercises are simple. Simple doesn't mean easy. The training routines in this book are tough to do. Don't let the hardship to discourage you. As you keep knocking down the training sessions one by one, you will not only get physically stronger but also you will get mentally stronger.

CHAPTER 5: PROGRESSIVE OVERLOAD

If you always put limit on everything you do, physical or anything else. It will spread into your work and into your life. There are no limits. There are only plateaus, and you must not stay there, you must go beyond them.

– Bruce Lee

If you want to get stronger, you need to progressively overload the stress you put on your muscles. If you do the same training over and over, you will remain the same. If you gradually increase the stress on your muscles, you will get stronger. This process is called progressive overload.

How To Apply Progressive Overload To Bodyweight Training

Progressive overload with weight training is straightforward. You increase the weight you are lifting or you increase the reps you do with the same weight.

With bodyweight training, you can't increase the weight you are lifting (as long as you don't get fat and I assume you don't want that) since you train with your own body's weight. In fact, you are going to lose fat during this program unless you are already slim.

With the routines in this book, there are 3 ways to achieve progressive overload:

1. **Increasing the number of reps.**
2. **Progressing to the proper version of the exercises.**
3. **Shortening the workout time.**

Increasing The Number Of Reps

Those of you who follow the beginner and intermediate routines will find their rep numbers increasing after the first 6 weeks. This will help them achieve progressive overload with their training. Those of you who follow the main routine will already be training with a high volume of reps, so you can't achieve progressive overload by increasing the rep numbers. You will still progress by applying the below methods.

Progressing To The Proper Version Of The Exercises

If you aren't already muscular and lean before you start the routines in this book, chances are that you will not be able to do all the exercises in their proper form. Not being able to start with the proper form of a specific exercise is not a problem, in fact, it's expected. If this is the case, you will start by doing the easy version of the exercise and you will progress to the proper version by getting stronger with the reps you complete with the easier version.

Shortening The Workout Time

Completing the workouts in a shorter time than the previous session is a great way to achieve progressive overload with bodyweight training.

For example, let's say your workout has 30 push-ups, 30 sit-ups and 15 pull-ups in total. If you completed this workout in 15 minutes today, try to complete it in less than 15 minutes next time. Soon, you will see that the duration of your workouts will be shorter and shorter which will save you tremendous time.

When you are training with the main routine and you are able to do all the exercises in their proper forms during all your workouts, shortening the workout time is the only way to achieve progressive overload.

For example, the main routine has a workout where you will do as many as 200 push-ups in a training session. Increasing the rep number beyond 200 in order to achieve progressive overload will be inefficient. Instead, you will try to complete the workout faster.

Since this is a time-efficient method to get stronger, I call it *the beauty of bodyweight training*. When other people need more and more time to get the most out of their workout routines, bodyweight athletes get stronger and stronger as they complete their training in shorter and shorter times.

When you get to the point of completing a bodyweight training session which has a large number of reps (such as 200 push-ups and 100 pull-ups) in less than 20 minutes, you will not only have a terrific body but also you will laugh at people who grind on the treadmill for hours just to lose fat. Moreover, men who grind endlessly on a treadmill look weak but a bodyweight athlete who can do 100 burpees in 5 minutes will look like a fitness model.

When I tell people that I built my six pack abs by training less than 3 hours a week (on average), they don't believe me but when you start doing the routines in this book, you will see that it's the truth. Don't be surprised if you find yourself training for less than 3 hours per week after a few weeks of training and you get a better body than 99% percent of the human population.

The Importance Of Keeping A Training Journal

Keep a training journal for writing down your training completion times per workout. Also, take notes on whether you had to resort to the easier versions of the exercises. The ideal is to do all the exercises with the proper form and complete the workouts in a shorter time than the previous ones.

Keep in mind that you don't have to be setting PR's (personal records) with each session. Bad days happen. Setting PR's is relatively easier during the first weeks of your program but they will be harder and harder to come by as you progress. You may hit plateaus as you get closer and closer to your potential.

How To Push Through Plateaus

It's highly unlikely that you will hit plateaus within the first weeks of your training, but when you get closer to your potential, PR's are harder to come by.

First of all, if you are happy with your progress so far, hitting plateaus isn't a bad thing in itself. If you are sure that you followed the instructions in this book and you gave it your all, hitting plateaus here and there are the signs of getting closer your potential.

But, if you are nowhere near your physique goals but still hitting plateaus that you can't overcome, here are a few things to remember.

1. ARE YOU SLEEPING ENOUGH?

If you aren't sleeping enough, it will hurt your training. Your muscles need to recover from your training and sleeping is the best way to recover. If you are sure that you are getting enough sleep, move on to the next item.

2. IS YOUR DIET EFFICIENT?

If you are gaining fat, this will harm your training performance as you are lifting an unnecessary additional weight with each rep you are doing. To know whether you are gaining fat or not isn't as easy as hopping on a scale and seeing whether the number is going up since you might as well be gaining more muscle than the fat you burn. Yes, it's possible to gain weight and still lose fat. For further information on learning your body fat percentage, refer to the Diet Chapter.

If you are on a plateau and you noticed that you are gaining fat, that's the cause of your plateau. Try losing fat by following the guidelines in the Diet Chapter.

Another problem with your diet may be that you are eating too little. While you certainly don't need to eat a ton of calories (and you shouldn't) for a better training performance, eating too little will also hurt your performance. If you don't get enough fuel from food, your training will suffer. If this is the case, try upping your calories by following the guidelines in the Diet Chapter.

Eating low-quality food, drinking too much alcohol, and smoking will all hurt your training performance, so keep these in mind when you find yourself hitting plateaus too soon too often.

Eating less than enough carbs, fat or protein will also hinder your progress, so I recommend you to monitor your food intake to make the necessary adjustments detailed in the Diet Chapter.

3. OTHER REASONS

Sometimes you may not be motivated enough to train or your mind will play tricks on you during your training which will hurt your performance.

The mind is extremely important in training. If your mind

doesn't want to train, your body will not train. When you find yourself mentally weak to push through when the going gets tough, read the chapter about muscle building mindset again. It's crucial to break the mental barriers as you will not progress otherwise.

CHAPTER 6: MUSCLE BUILDING, FAT BURNING DIET

The only way you get that fat off is to eat less and exercise more.

-Jack LaLanne

For muscle building purposes, there's nothing more important than your training. When I started bodyweight training I didn't know the best way to eat, so I ended up eating too much that I failed to lose body fat for a long time. But on the plus side, I got strong because I trained hard. I wish I knew what I knew now about diet because I would have reached my physique goals a lot earlier.

The diet techniques you will learn in these chapters are the result of years of trial and error so you are lucky to know them from the start. If you understand that training isn't enough for burning fat (even when you train hard), half the battle is won. You must care about your diet if you want to get lean.

Diet is the most essential part of burning fat and it's also important for building muscle. There's a fine line between eating enough food to fuel your training and not going overboard and gain weight.

Obviously, how much you will be eating during the program

depends on your current physical condition. If you are starting overweight, you will eat less and if you are starting underweight you will eat more.

Let's first go over the basics and then let's find out what and how much you will eat during your training.

Determining Your Diet Goals

If you follow the guidelines in this book and stick to your workout routine, you will build muscle. However, whether you want to lose fat depends on your current body fat level.

If you want to have visible six pack abs, you will have to be at 8-10% body fat level. If you just want a fit looking body but you don't care about six-pack abs, getting to 12-15% body fat will be enough to achieve your goal. When your body fat percentage goes up to the north of 15%, you start to look fat. So, I don't recommend it. If you currently have more 15% body fat, you will probably want to lose fat. If you are already below 15% of body fat, whether you want to gain fat, keep your current body fat levels or lose fat will depend on your physique goals.

Before we get into the details of your diet, let's find out your current body fat percentage.

How To Determine Your Body Fat Percentage

You can measure your body fat percentage with a skinfold caliper. Alternatively, a bioelectrical impedance body composition monitor can give you a good idea about your body fat percentage too. A DEXA scan can give you an exact number but I don't recommend you to obsess over your exact body fat percentage.

The problem with the above methods for measuring your body fat percentage is that they all will give you a different number. They are good for tracking your progress once you determine a benchmark and you are consistent with your measuring method, but there's an easier way.

You can take a shirtless picture or look at your body in the mirror and guess your body fat percentage. Here's a picture for reference:

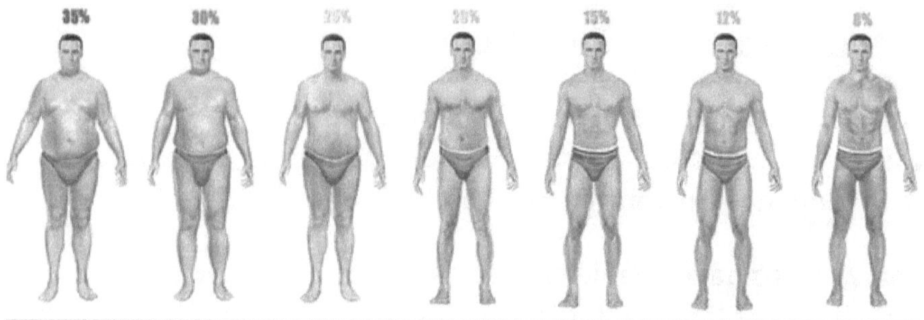

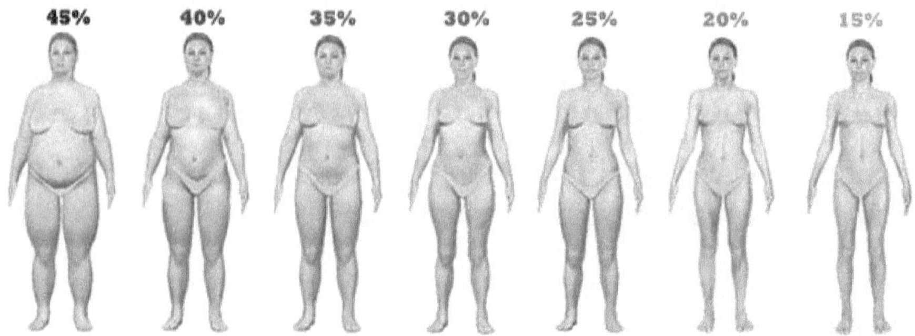

Just by looking at your body in the mirror or a picture, you will know whether you want to lose fat or not.

Weight Loss (Or Gain) Depends On How Many Calories You Eat

The fitness industry is working hard to make you believe that calories don't matter for fat loss so that they can sell all kinds of bullshit products to gullible people who want an easy way to lose fat (which doesn't exist, by the way).

In reality, weight loss is all about eating fewer calories than you burn and weight gain is about eating more calories than you burn. It's always been this way and it will always be. Food is essentially energy. The first law of thermodynamics, also known as the Law of Conservation of Energy, states that energy cannot be created or destroyed in an isolated system. You can't break the laws of nature.

You lose weight by eating fewer calories than you burn and you gain weight by eating more calories than you burn. Period.

Predicting Your Daily Calorie Expenditure

Your daily calorie expenditure gives you the number of calories you should eat to maintain your body weight. Always remember that your body composition may change even when you are maintaining your weight depending on the nutritional value of the calories you consume and your daily activities.

If you are sedentary and eat a lot of carbs or drink too much alcohol, you will lose muscle mass and gain body fat even when you consume maintenance calories and your body weight doesn't change. On the contrary, when you are training for strength and eating enough protein, fat, and carbs, you will lose fat and gain muscle even though you eat at maintenance calories and your weight doesn't change.

Also, keep in mind that your daily calorie expenditure changes as your weight, body composition, and activity levels change. Your daily calorie expenditure isn't set in stone, so remember to calculate it regularly if you are counting your calories.

You can use a calorie calculator for a fairly accurate guess at https://tdeecalculator.net/. (Choose the moderate exercise option as you will be training 4 times a week.)

How Many Calories A Day Should You Eat?

Depending on whether you want to lose fat or not, you should adjust your calorie and macro intake according to your goals.

If you want to lose fat and gain muscle at the same time, it's best for you to eat fewer calories than you burn and adjust your protein, fat, and carb intake. You can lose fat and gain muscle at the same time by eating at maintenance calories but if your aim is to get lean and strong as fast as possible, it's not the best strategy to use.

The trick here is to not eat so little that you fail to build muscle and not eat so much that you gain fat. It's possible to gain muscle and lose fat at the same time, as long as you stick to your training routine and eat according to your daily calorie and macro goals.

First, let's look at how many calories a day you should eat in order to lose fat without stunting your muscle gains. Find your body fat percentage and your daily calorie expenditure according to the guidelines above and determine the daily caloric deficit you must create by the corresponding row on the chart below:

Your Body Fat %	Average Daily Caloric Deficit You Need to Create
30+%	700+ calories
26-30%	600 calories
22-25%	500 calories
18-21%	400 calories
15-17%	300 calories

13-14%   250 calories

Note that this the *average* daily caloric deficit you must create. You don't need to create the same deficit day in day out. As long as you keep the average, you will be fine. For example, let's say you are at 18-21% body fat and you are looking at a daily caloric deficit of 500 calories. Creating a deficit of 600 calories one day and 400 calories the next day is perfectly fine. You may even eat a surplus of calories on some days and go below your average daily deficit on other days to maintain your average deficit. For the exact number of macros to eat, refer to the macro breakdown section below. If you have more than 30% of body fat, you can eat at a caloric deficit that is more than 700 but you should be careful about your training. If you can at least perform the easier version of the exercises, you can train.

If you are already lean and you don't want to lose fat, you must eat at your maintenance calories.

If you are too skinny and you want to gain fat, you must eat more than your maintenance calories. How many more calories you should eat depends on how much weight you want to gain. Eat at a 5-10% of caloric surplus if you want to minimize fat gain and maximize muscle gain. Eating more than that will result in unwanted and unnecessary fat gain.

How To Gain Weight (If You Are Too Skinny)

There are many people who swear that they eat a lot but they are unable to gain weight. That's impossible unless you have a thyroid malfunction in which case you should see a doctor. In most situations, skinny people who are unable to gain weight overestimate the calories they consume. Find out your daily calorie expenditure with the method mentioned above and count your calories to make sure you are eating more calories than you burn. You will see that you will start to gain weight when you eat at a caloric surplus.

Macros

A calorie is a calorie in the realm of weight change but since you will be building muscle, weight loss or weight gain doesn't mean too much to you. You must focus on fat loss instead of weight loss and muscle gain instead of weight gain. For example, if you build 10 pounds of muscle and lose 10 pounds of fat during your program, you will weigh exactly the same as you started but you will be a lot fitter and stronger.

So, for muscle building and nutritional purposes, you have to take your macros into account, i.e. where your calories are coming from. Not all calories are the same in terms of nutritional value.

There are 2 kinds of nutrients. Macronutrients and micronutrients. Macro is a short-term for macronutrients.

There are 3 kinds of macros:

- **Proteins** (~4 calories per gram)
- **Fats** (~ 9 calories per gram)
- **Carbohydrates** (Also known as carbs) (~ 4 calories per gram)

Micronutrients are vitamins and minerals. They don't have calories.

Warning: There is one more substance that contains calories: Alcohol.

Alcohol is neither a macronutrient nor a micronutrient. Alcohol contains 7 calories per gram but it has no nutritional value. I don't recommend alcohol during your program. If you have to drink, keep it moderate and be aware that alcohol calories

COUNT.

Macro Breakdown: How Much Protein, Fat, And Carbs You Should Eat

HOW MUCH PROTEIN SHOULD YOU EAT?

First, you must eat your animal protein. Eating enough animal protein will accomplish a few things:

When you are building muscle (and burning fat), you need to keep your existing muscles and add muscle mass to your body. Protein is the building block of muscles. So, you need to eat protein.

If you are losing fat, being in a caloric deficit when you are training hard will be tough. Trust me, you will feel hungry. Protein is the most satiating macronutrient. Eating more protein will make you feel less hungry.

Protein has a thermic effect. Your metabolism will slow down when you are in a caloric deficit. Protein will help increase your metabolic rate.

To build muscle, you need to eat at least 0.8 grams of protein per pound of your body weight. When you are in a caloric deficit, you need to eat even more protein than that. While you are training and dieting for fat loss, eat 1-1.2 grams of protein per pound of your body weight every day.

HOW MUCH FAT SHOULD YOU EAT?

Fat is an essential nutrient. You need to eat fat to keep your hormones in check. Fat being essential doesn't mean you need to be eating too much though. If you want to lose body fat, eat 0.2-0.3 grams of fat per pound of your body weight every day. If you not aiming to lose fat, you can increase your fat intake according to your daily calorie goals.

HOW MUCH CARBS SHOULD YOU EAT?

Carbohydrates (AKA Carbs) are not essential for survival but you need to eat them when you are training hard.

Carbs will provide quick energy for your training sessions.

On non-training days, you still need to eat carbs to avoid ketosis. Long-term effects of ketosis are not understood yet, so it's better to be safe than sorry.

If you are targeting fat loss, eat 1-1.2 gram of carbs per pound of your body weight on your training days. Eat approximately 100 gr of carbs to avoid ketosis on your rest days.

If you are not targeting fat loss you can increase your carb intake according to your daily calorie goals.

Protein Sources

Eggs, egg whites, beef, lamb, pork, chicken, turkey, fish, squid, shrimp, cheese, yogurt, and milk are all excellent protein sources.

If you are targeting fat loss, eat lean cuts of meat, cottage cheese, low-fat yogurt and skim milk.

I mostly ate eggs, beef, chicken, and tuna during my fat loss diet. You can choose your favorite animal protein source.

Warning: If you are targeting fat loss, it's essential to understand that different cuts of meat have different fat content. Since you won't have a generous calorie budget, aim for lean cuts of meat. See the table below to have an idea of how different parts of an animal have different content of fat and calories.

Food	Protein (gr)	Fat (gr)	Carb (gr)	Calories
Beef Lean (100 gr)	24.1	5.0	0.0	152.0
Beef Tenderloin (Lean Only, Trimmed to 1/8" Fat) (100 gr)	22.1	6.5	0.0	152.0
Beef Ribeye (100 gr)	16.0	15.1	0.0	200.0
Ground Beef (%5 fat) (100 gr)	21.0	5.0	0.0	136.0
Ground Beef (%10 fat) (100 gr)	20.0	10.0	0.0	176.0
Ground Lamb (100 gr)	17.0	23.0	0.0	282.0
Chicken Breast (100 gr)	31.0	3.6	0.0	165.0
Chicken Breast with skin (100 gr)	29.5	7.4	0.0	180.0
Chicken Leg with Bone and Skin	13.2	5.9	0.0	110.0
Tuna 180 gr can in water	33.0	0.0	0.0	120.0
Squid (100 gr)	16.0	1.4	3.1	92.0
Pork ribs with bone (100 gr)	15.8	8.0	3.1	175.0
Egg (1 large 50 gr)	6.0	5.0	0.6	78.0
Egg White (1 large 33 gr)	3.6	0.1	0.2	17.0

Also, note that egg whites have significantly lower calories than whole eggs. That's because egg yolks contain fat and egg whites don't.

Fat Sources

You will inevitably eat some fat from your animal protein sources.

In addition, you can add some butter, olive oil, fish oil, flaxseed oil or coconut oil to your diet.

If you are targeting fat loss, you don't have too much of a fat budget so use it carefully since it's too easy to eat too many calories from fat as one gram of fat contains a whopping 9 calories.

I prefer to mix eggs and egg whites to avoid eating too many calories from fat. Eggs have their fat content in the yolk so egg whites will not hurt you. 4 egg whites and 1 whole egg can make a fairly tasty omelet.

Carb Sources

Fruits, vegetables, potatoes, rice, pasta, wheat, oats are all good sources of carbs, as long as you don't exceed your calorie budget.

I find potatoes more filling than pasta, wheat or rice but that's just me. Choose the carb source of your liking and don't go over your calorie budget.

Try to mix your carb sources. Potatoes, rice, pasta, wheat, oats contain starch. Fruits contain fructose. Vegetables are fiber-rich.

I prefer to eat potatoes, bananas, apples, tomatoes, cucumber, radish and lettuce for my carb requirements.

Vegetables are low in calorie content so it's a good idea to eat lots of vegetables. Some vegetables can have too many calories so be sure to include those calories in your calorie budget.

Eating vegetables will help you suppress your hunger with relatively lower calories. They will also add color and flavor to your meals. There's a lot to love about vegetables, especially when you are on a fat loss diet. Use them to your advantage.

Sample Daily Meal Plan For Fat Loss

Here's my typical daily fat loss diet:

Breakfast: 5 egg whites (85 calories), 1 whole egg (78 calories), 3 small size tomatoes (33 calories), 1 medium-sized banana (90 calories)

Lunch: 300 grams of chicken breast (495 calories), 300 grams of potatoes (231 calories), vegetable salad with tomatoes, cucumber and radish (80 calories), 1 medium-sized apple (84 calories)

Dinner: 300 grams of 5% fat ground beef (408 calories), 200 grams of potatoes (154 calories), lettuce salad with olive oil (155 calories), 1 medium-sized banana (90 calories)

Total: 1983 calories (200 gr protein, 47 gr fat, 187 gr carbs)

Note that I was around 15% of body fat when I ate like this. Adjust your macros and calories according to the caloric deficit table above.

My Tips About Fat Loss

Being in a caloric deficit while you are training hard is difficult.

Here are my tips to make it easier:

Tip #1: Learn to cook a few delicious meals. An oven, a grill or a slow cooker can do wonders for cooking low calorie, high nutrient dishes. Try them.

Tip #2: Coffee suppresses hunger and has zero calories. Drink some black coffee when you feel hungry.

Tip #3: Use condiments to add color and flavor to your meals. Sprinkling some black pepper, chili, cumin etc. on your meals makes them tastier. You can also add low-calorie sauces such as salsa.

Tip #4: Remember that this is temporary. Cravings are your body's tricks to make you eat more calories. Maintaining your body fat percentage is easy once you get to the point you want. It pays to be patient until you get there.

Frequently Asked Questions About Diet

ISN'T TRAINING ENOUGH? WHY SHOULD I DIET?

You can't out-train your diet. Training doesn't burn as many calories as you think.

HOW MANY MEALS A DAY SHOULD I EAT?

Hitting your macro (protein, fat, and carbohydrates) goals and the total number of calories you eat is all that matters. I eat 2-3 meals a day but you can eat as often as you want as long as you don't exceed your daily average calorie goals. Meal timing doesn't affect fat loss or gain.

WILL IT HURT ME IF I EAT AT NIGHT?

No. When I'm on diet, I prefer eating close to my sleep time because I can't sleep when I'm hungry. The calories you eat is what matters. Not the time of the day you eat them.

IS PROTEIN SHAKE OK?

Yes. Just check the carb and fat content of your protein powder and count those calories too.

WHAT ABOUT CHEAT MEALS?

You can eat cheat meals here and there but don't forget to count your calories. You will be fine as long as you don't exceed your calorie budget.

DO I NEED TO EAT THE VEGETABLES RAW OR COOKED?

Whichever you like.

CAN I EAT CANNED TUNA?

Yes.

CAN I EAT OR DRINK EGGS WITH EVERY MEAL?

Yes.

CAN I USE SALT?

Yes.

CAN I EAT NUTS?

I don't recommend nuts for fat loss because they are too high in calories. If you must eat them, don't exceed your daily calorie budget.

I HAVE A FLAT STOMACH BUT NO ABS. IS THIS NORMAL?

Yes. Your ab muscles are still muscles so you need to train and build them too. The routines in this book will build your ab muscles.

DO I NEED SUPPLEMENTS?

I take vitamin D and fish oil semi-regularly but it's dubious whether they help with anything or not.

DO YOU HAVE ANY SUGGESTIONS FOR WHAT TO EAT BEFORE OR AFTER WORKOUTS?

Eating your carbs 2 hours before your training may improve your training performance. Everybody reacts differently to pre-workout feeding so your best bet is to try different methods to see what works the best for you.

CAN I DRINK SPORTS DRINKS?

Hydration is an essential part of training so I always recommend drinking plenty of water before, during and after your training. You can replace water with a sports drink but don't forget to count those calories.

CHAPTER 7: TRAINING GUIDELINES

The last three or four reps is what makes the muscle grow. This area of pain divides the champion from someone else who is not a champion. That's what most people lack, having the guts to go on and just say they'll go through the pain no matter what happens.

– Arnold Schwarzenegger

Before we get into the workouts, we will look at the training guidelines which will help you to get the most out of your training sessions.

Training Frequency

You will train 4 times per week. You will train hard and you will need the rest days. 3 days for resting is enough for recovery provided that you follow the recovery techniques provided in this chapter.

It's best to distribute the rest days between training days. For example, you can choose to train on Monday, Tuesday, Thursday, and Saturday and rest on Wednesday, Friday, and Sunday. Or you can train on Monday, Wednesday, Friday, and Sunday and rest on Tuesday, Thursday, and Saturday.

There will inevitably be at least 2 consecutive days of training in a week but don't worry about that. I designed the routines in a way to avoid overtraining.

Training Volume

I fixed the training volume of the main routine for the purposes of maximum muscle growth with minimum time investment, which means that the rep numbers will not change as you progress with your training but your training time will decrease as you get better.

You will achieve progressive overload by completing the workouts faster than your previous workouts. Don't forget to keep a training journal to write down how long it took you to complete a particular workout so that you are able to know whether you are progressing or not. Progressing means you are improving your endurance and body composition (more muscle, less fat). Also, don't forget to take shirtless pictures before you start your routine and keep taking pictures regularly (for example, once a week) to see your progress.

The rep numbers may appear too many at the beginning but you will quickly get used to doing them and your training time will get shorter and shorter.

I included a beginner and and intermediate routine for those of you who may be discouraged by the difficulty of the main routine. The beginner and intermediate routines start with lower volume and the volume increases by week 6.

Training Session Length

There's no fixed training session length. Your training session ends when you complete doing all the reps within your session.

In the beginning, it may take you a while to complete your sessions but your body will be quick to adapt provided that you sleep and eat properly.

Even for the main routine where the rep numbers are the highest, you can expect to cut your training time below a total of 3 hours a week after a few weeks of training, and as you progress, don't be surprised when you train for only 2 hours in a week and have a body better than 99% of the population.

If you are doing the beginner or intermediate routines, you can expect to finish the workouts quicker as you will be doing fewer reps than the ones who are following the main routine.

Warm Up

You can warm up by doing 5-10 controlled reps for each of the easy versions of the exercises in your workout.

Some light jogging and stretching will also be helpful to send blood to your muscles to warm them up before training.

Since you will train with your body weight, the risk of injury is low but it's best to be on the safe side and not skip your warm-up.

Rep Speed

Rep speed may be as fast as you want as long as you don't sacrifice proper form.

Don't try to slow down your reps thinking that this will build more muscle. It won't.

Think of it like real life. Do you consciously try to slow down in real life whenever you are using your muscles? If you are not doing it in real life, then it doesn't make sense to do it in your training. The muscles you build during your workouts will result in real-life functionality so your natural instinct to adjust your rep speed will do just fine.

The only exception to this rule is when you are doing negative pull-ups. The negative portion of the negative pull-ups should be slow and controlled.

> **Warning:** When you are doing regular pull-ups you don't need to slow down during the negative portion of the exercise. You only slow down in the negative portion of pull-ups when you are unable to do regular pull-ups and have to proceed with negative pull-ups.

Rest Intervals Between Sets And Fatigue Issues

There are no set rest intervals between sets. Ideally, it's best to complete the workouts without no rest intervals whatsoever but that will not be possible in real life because you will inevitably rest at times when you want to catch your breath or your muscles are too fatigued to continue.

Finish the workouts as fast as you can without breaking form. When you need to rest, rest enough until you can continue your workout. It doesn't matter how many sets it takes to complete your reps, even if it means you are doing sets of one rep by the end.

For example, let's say your workout schedule tells you to do 50 burpees. Doing 50 burpees in a row isn't possible unless you are an elite athlete, so you will do them by taking little breaks whenever you feel you can't continue anymore. Let's say you did 10 burpees and you are out of breath. Take a little break to catch your breath and when you are ready, do 10 more burpees. If you can't do another 10, do 7, 5, 3 or 1. Keep on like this until you complete all the reps.

If you are too fatigued and you can no longer do the full version of the exercises, proceed with the easy version of the particular exercise that you can't do anymore. The easy versions of the exercises are provided in the Exercises Chapter. If you can't even do the easier version of a particular exercise, rest as long as you can until you can at least do the easy version. Unless you are injured, never quit your workout prematurely.

Completing all the reps in your training session is of utmost importance. If you quit before you finish doing all your reps, you sabotage your efforts. Always remember that your muscles grow the most during the last few reps. Think of all the other reps before the last round as a preparation for the real thing. If you quit before doing the last reps, you will have trained in vain. Remember, quitters aren't winners and winners aren't quitters.

Number Of Reps Used

The number of reps used is high as you will be training with only your bodyweight. Don't let the high number of reps to intimidate you because you will see that your body will be quick to adapt to the training volume and intensity. Muscles grow by adaptation. If you don't put enough stress on your muscles, they will not grow. It's not possible to exert enough stress on your body by doing a few reps with bodyweight exercises.

You will not get anywhere by doing 2 pull-ups here, 3 push-ups there. Since you can't increase the weight you are lifting with each bodyweight exercise, you have no option other than increasing the number of reps. On the other hand, you can't increase the number of reps beyond a particular number because who has the time for doing, for example, 600 push-ups?

As a result, I fixed the rep numbers for the main routine to a reasonably high number (but not too high to take an unnecessarily long time) and I distributed the reps for each exercise between the reps of other exercises so that you will practically be supersetting between your selected exercises for any workout.

Measuring Your Progress

You measure your progress by noting down the time it takes to complete a particular session. If you complete the same session faster than before, it means that you are progressing. Progress means that you are losing fat, building muscle or gaining endurance. Most of the time, these 3 factors are all happening at the same time provided that you are watching your diet.

Another progress you may achieve is to complete more of the exercises with the full version. You may resort to doing the easier versions of some exercises, especially at the beginning of your program, but as you get stronger, you will notice that you are able to do more and more of the full versions of the exercises. When you are doing your workouts, note it down when you resort to the easier version of a particular exercise. When you do the same workout in the future and do more reps of the full version of that particular exercise, it means that you progressed.

When you get better and better (and you will), you will see that your workouts are taking you less and less time to complete. Ideally, you get to a point where you finish all your workout sessions in less than 30 minutes, so your weekly total time of training goes below 2 hours.

Techniques For Recovery

Your workouts are intense so it's essential to recover from your training.

You already have 3 days for recovery which I think is more than enough. As a general rule, you must always get enough sleep. Sleep is essential for recovery as you will sabotage your efforts when you don't sleep enough to allow your body to recover for your next training session. I sleep 7-8 hours a day but sleep schedules will differ according to your build. If you feel the need to nap during the daytime, that's a good indicator of not getting enough night's sleep. Ideally, you should get enough sleep at night to not need to nap but if you must nap before a workout then it's better to nap than not to nap and do a poor workout.

Alcohol and sleep pills hurt the quality of sleep, so it's best to avoid them for a full recovery. If you must drink then drink moderately. Heavy drinking will hurt your progress.

Your muscles will get sore especially at the beginning. I personally ignore the muscle soreness and proceed with my training as scheduled. Muscle soreness might be an issue for the first few weeks of your program but it should subside after a few weeks. If soreness bothers you too much, you can get a deep tissue massage.

Injury Prevention

Don't skip your warm-ups before your training sessions.

If you feel pain in or have trouble moving a particular body part or, don't ignore it. It may signal an injury. If the problem persists see a specialist.

Don't break proper form while you are doing your exercises. Bad form is often the result of an inability to perform the exercises with a proper form. If this is the case, proceed to do the exercises with the easier versions. Other times, you may compromise form in the name of scoring new personal bests. Don't do this. Honesty is always a key to physical and mental development.

Hydration

High-intensity bodyweight exercises will make you sweat. Keep a bottle of water with you while you are training. Sports drinks are also an option. I frequently drink them while I am training.

Be careful about drinking too much alcohol. Alcohol dehydrates you. It's best to avoid it altogether but if you must drink then drink lots of water the next day to stay hydrated.

Workout Clothes, Shoes, Gear

Wear comfortable clothing that doesn't limit your mobility.

Working out without shoes is perfectly fine. Since I do bodyweight training mostly at home I don't wear shoes while training. If you are working out in a gym or outside, flat sole sports shoes are better.

You don't need any gear for bodyweight workouts. I don't wear gloves while doing pull-ups but I am not against it. Getting results is what matters. If you have the body of a Greek god, nobody cares whether you wore gloves while doing pull-ups or you did them with your bare hands.

The Best Time To Work Out

The best time to work out is the time that fits your schedule. In other words, there's no set in stone best time to work out. I prefer to work out well into the afternoon or early in the evening, a time when I am finished with the day's work. I don't think the time to work out will change the results you get from training.

I also don't think whether you are feeling good, bad, tired, or rested will have a significant effect on your workouts. I had some of my best workouts when I was feeling tired, worn out from a day of hard work, or when I was feeling down. I also had some of my worst workouts when I was well rested, feeling great and ready to break records. You don't really know how your workout will turn out before you actually start training.

Many people make the mistake of skipping training when they are feeling down. It should be the opposite. There are not so many better ways than a strength training workout to uplift your mood. Strength training is proven to increase the release of the happy hormones in your brain. There have been many times when I started to train while feeling down and I ended up feeling great after I finished training. Don't let your mood manipulate you.

How To Spot Your Brain Trying To Trick You

The human body doesn't like being driven out of its comfort zone, so your brain will play tricks on you to skip the day's training and do something comfortable.

"Come on let's skip training and watch TV/play video games/drink beer/go out and have fun"

"Let's skip the training for today. You will do it tomorrow."

This is your brain trying to talk you out of training. Because it doesn't like discomfort. Ignore his antics and proceed with your training.

"Come on, you trained enough, let's just finish it here."

"Why did you get yourself into this? Life can still be good when you are not in great shape. Come on this is too tough. You are not a professional athlete. Let's quit it here."

"Oh no, not another 50 reps of burpees. Let's quit, I am already tired."

This is your brain trying to sabotage the training session you already started. It wants you to go back to the comfort zone. Always remember that quitters aren't winners and winners aren't quitters. Proceed with your training until you finish your planned workout.

CHAPTER 8: THE WORKOUTS & THE ROUTINES

When the going gets tough, the tough get going.

-Joseph Kennedy

There are 10 different workouts that you will be doing over and over throughout your preferred routine. I designed all the workouts in a way that they can be done in circuits ranging from one to five. Every workout represents one circuit which stands on its own. As for the routines in this book, doing one circuit of a particular workout is the easiest and doing five circuits is the most difficult.

There are 3 types of routines:

1. Beginner routine → *1 to 2 circuits of each workout*
2. Intermediate routine → *3 to 4 circuits of each workout*
3. The main routine → *5 circuits of each workout*

I named the routines as "beginner", "intermediate" and "the main" only for the sake of convenience. I say convenience because I believe that every one of you can skip the beginner and intermediate routines and start right from the main routine from day 1, no matter what your athletic background is.

However, I am aware of the fact that not everybody will be able to start from the main routine, not because they can't do it but because, in the beginning, it's tough to handle the intensity of the main routine.

In the past few years, many of my friends and family members asked me about my bodyweight workout routine. I used to give them my routine and they would start training. Some of them were unable to complete their first workout and quit training altogether because they were intimidated by the intensity. I noticed that if I give them an option for an easier routine to get their feet wet, they are more likely to continue training. This is the reason I decided to include beginner and intermediate routines in this book. Bodyweight training is so beneficial that I don't want any of you to get discouraged and quit by day 1.

Obviously, the main routine is where the greatest gains happen. As I said, you can start directly from the main routine. I see no problem with that. If the main routine is too much too soon for you, you can start with the beginner or intermediate routines and build up from there. Additionally, not everyone wants a ripped body with six-pack abs. If that's you, the beginner or the intermediate routines are capable of building you decent muscle mass.

The beginner routine starts with one circuit of the workouts for the first 6 weeks and continues with two circuits after the week 6.

The intermediate routine starts with three circuits of the workouts for the first 6 weeks and continues with four circuits after the week 6.

The main routine starts and ends with five circuits of all workouts throughout the whole 12 weeks.

If you start with the beginner or intermediate routines and decide to continue with the main routine before you finish your current routine, you can do so by jumping to the first week of the main routine.

If you start with the main routine as I urge you to do, don't be discouraged if you can't do the full versions of all the exercises in your workout. Completing all the exercises in a workout with their fully proper form takes time, so just keep going by doing the easier versions of the exercises you have trouble doing properly. Same goes for the beginner and intermediate routines.

The most important part of the routines is to complete all your reps. Don't worry if you can't do the full versions of the exercises. Keep doing the easier versions until you build enough strength to complete them with their full versions. The full and easier versions of the exercises can be found at the Exercises Chapter.

Let's first look at the workouts and then we will proceed to the routines.

The Workouts

All workouts represent a circuit of a group of exercises which should be completed in the order they appear.

- If you are following the beginner routine, you will do the circuit only once for the first 6 weeks and twice from week 7 on.
- If you are following the intermediate routine you will repeat the circuit three times for the first 6 weeks and four times after the week 7.
- If you are following the main routine you will repeat the circuit five times throughout the whole 12 weeks.

For example, for the *Upper Body Strength* workout below, those of you who are following the beginner routine will first do 15 pull-ups, then do 30 push-ups, and then do 30 sit-ups and you are finished with your training session. Your session will look like:

- 15 pull-ups/ 30 push-ups/ 30 sit-ups → *1 Circuit*

Your workload will increase to 2 circuits after the week 6.

If you are following the intermediate routine, you will do 3 circuits of the same workout for the first six weeks of your routine. Your training session for the *Upper Body Strength* workout will look like:

- 15 pull-ups/ 30 push-ups/ 30 sit-ups → *1ˢᵗ Circuit*
- 15 pull-ups/ 30 push-ups/ 30 sit-ups → *2ⁿᵈ Circuit*
- 15 pull-ups/ 30 push-ups/ 30 sit-ups → *3ʳᵈ Circuit*

Your workload will increase to 4 circuits after the week 6.

If you are following the main routine, you will do 5 circuits of the same workout. Your training session for the *Upper Body Strength* workout will look like:

- 15 pull-ups/ 30 push-ups/ 30 sit-ups → *1ˢᵗ Circuit*
- 15 pull-ups/ 30 push-ups/ 30 sit-ups → *2ⁿᵈ Circuit*
- 15 pull-ups/ 30 push-ups/ 30 sit-ups → *3ʳᵈ Circuit*
- 15 pull-ups/ 30 push-ups/ 30 sit-ups → *4ᵗʰ Circuit*
- 15 pull-ups/ 30 push-ups/ 30 sit-ups → *5ᵗʰ Circuit*

You will always do 5 circuits of all the workouts for the whole 12 weeks. You will progress by completing his workouts faster or doing more of the proper form of the exercises.

There are no mandatory breaks between the reps and the circuits. For example, those of you who are following the main routine and doing the *Upper Body Strength* workout for the day can proceed to your next 15 pull-ups, right after you finish the 30 sit-ups at the end of your first circuit.

Complete the given number of exercises no matter how many sets it takes even if it means doing sets of one rep by the end. For example, when you are doing the 15 pull-ups in the *Upper Body Strength* workout, you can start by doing 5 reps of pull-ups, then take a small break until you catch your breath or allow for your muscles to get ready for more reps. You can do 3 more reps and take another break, 2 more reps and take another break and so on. If you are no longer able to do the full version of a given exercise, proceed with the easier version. All the reps of all the exercises in a given workout must be completed even if it means you must resort to the easier version of a particular exercise.

I named the workouts for the dominant muscle groups trained but since you will be doing compound exercises, there will always be other muscle groups trained with all the workouts you do.

Here are the workouts:

UPPER BODY STRENGTH

- 15 pull-ups
- 30 push-ups
- 30 sit-ups

CORE STRENGTH

- 15 burpees
- 30 sit-ups
- 15 burpees
- 20 lunges

FRONTAL STRENGTH

- 20 push-ups
- 40 squats
- 20 push-ups
- 20 sit-ups

LEGS STRENGTH

- 50 lunges
- 10 jumps
- 50 squats
- 10 jumps

V-TAPER

- 20 burpees
- 10 pull-ups
- 20 push-ups
- 30 squats

FULL-FLEDGED STRENGTH

- 15 pull-ups
- 30 push-ups
- 30 sit-ups
- 30 squats

EXPLOSIVE STRENGTH

- 30 burpees
- 7 pull-ups
- 15 push-ups

UPPER BODY SKILLS

- 7 pull-ups
- 14 push-ups
- 21 sit-ups

CORE SKILLS

- 20 burpees
- 10 jumps

LEGS SKILLS

- 20 squats
- 20 lunges
- 20 leg raises

Workouts At A Glance

CORE STRENGTH	FULL-FLEDGED STRENGTH	LEGS STRENGTH
15x Burpees	15x Pull-ups	50x Lunges
30x Sit-ups	30x Push-ups	10x Jumps
15x Burpees	30x Sit-ups	50x Squats
20x Lunges	30x Squats	10x Jumps

V-TAPER	FRONTAL STRENGTH	UPPER BODY STRENGTH
20x Burpees	20x Push-ups	15x Pull-ups
10x Pull-ups	40x Squats	30x Push-ups
20x Push-ups	20x Push-ups	30x Sit-ups
30x Squats	20x Sit-ups	

LEGS SKILLS	EXPLOSIVE STRENGTH	UPPER BODY SKILLS
20x Squats	30x Burpees	7x Pull-ups
20x Lunges	7x Pull-ups	14x Push-ups
20x Leg Raises	15x Push-ups	21x Sit-ups

CORE SKILLS		
20x Burpees		
10x Jumps		

The Routines

There are 3 routines which are classified as beginner, intermediate, and the main. The workout order is the same for all the routines. The difference is only in the volume.

The workload for the beginner and the intermediate routines will increase after the week 6 as you will be more comfortable with the exercises after 6 weeks of training. The workload for the main routine will stay the same for 12 weeks as you will already be training with the highest volume. You will progress by completing the workouts faster and doing more of the proper form of the exercises. Those of you who are following the beginner and the intermediate routines will progress by volume, workout completion time and doing more of the proper version of the exercises.

The Beginner Routine

	Day 1	Day 2	Day 3	Day 4
Week 1	Frontal Strength	Core Strength	Upper Body Skills	Explosive Strength
Week 2	Core Strength	V-Taper	Legs Skills	Frontal Strength
Week 3	Upper Body Skills	Explosive Strength	Core Skills	Full-Fledged Strength
Week 4	Frontal Strength	Upper Body Skills	Explosive Strength	Legs Skills
Week 5	Upper Body Strength	Legs Strength	Upper Body Skills	Full-Fledged Strength
Week 6	V-Taper	Legs Skills	Frontal Strength	Upper Body Strength
Week 7	Core Skills x 2	Frontal Strength x 2	Legs Strength x 2	Upper Body Skills x 2
Week 8	Explosive Strength x 2	Frontal Strength x 2	Core Strength x 2	Frontal Strength x 2
Week 9	Legs Strength x 2	V-Taper x 2	Core Skills x 2	Full-Fledged Strength x 2
Week 10	Core Strength x 2	Upper Body Skills x 2	Core Strength x 2	Full-Fledged Strength x 2
Week 11	Legs Strength x 2	V-Taper x 2	Core Skills x 2	Upper Body Strength x 2
Week 12	Explosive Strength x 2	Core Strength x 2	V-Taper x 2	Frontal Strength x 2

The Intermediate Routine

	Day 1	Day 2	Day 3	Day 4
Week 1	Frontal Strength x 3	Core Strength x 3	Upper Body Skills x 3	Explosive Strength x 3

	Day 1	Day 2	Day 3	Day 4
Week 2	Core Strength x 3	V-Taper x 3	Legs Skills x 3	Frontal Strength x 3
Week 3	Upper Body Skills x 3	Explosive Strength x 3	Core Skills x 3	Full-Fledged Strength x 3
Week 4	Frontal Strength x 3	Upper Body Skills x 3	Explosive Strength x 3	Legs Skills x 3
Week 5	Upper Body Strength x 3	Legs Strength x 3	Upper Body Skills x 3	Full-Fledged Strength x 3
Week 6	V-Taper x 3	Legs Skills x 3	Frontal Strength x 3	Upper Body Strength x 3
Week 7	Core Skills x 4	Frontal Strength x 4	Legs Strength x 4	Upper Body Skills x 4
Week 8	Explosive Strength x 4	Frontal Strength x 4	Core Strength x 4	Frontal Strength x 4
Week 9	Legs Strength x 4	V-Taper x 4	Core Skills x 4	Full-Fledged Strength x 4
Week 10	Core Strength x 4	Upper Body Skills x 4	Core Strength x 4	Full-Fledged Strength x 4
Week 11	Legs Strength x 4	V-Taper x 4	Core Skills x 4	Upper Body Strength x 4
Week 12	Explosive Strength x 4	Core Strength x 4	V-Taper x 4	Frontal Strength x 4

The Main Routine

	Day 1	Day 2	Day 3	Day 4
Week 1	Frontal Strength x 5	Core Strength x 5	Upper Body Skills x 5	Explosive Strength x 5
Week 2	Core Strength x 5	V-Taper x 5	Legs Skills x 5	Frontal Strength x 5

Week 3	Upper Body Skills x 5	Explosive Strength x 5	Core Skills x 5	Full-Fledged Strength x 5
Week 4	Frontal Strength x 5	Upper Body Skills x 5	Explosive Strength x 5	Legs Skills x 5
Week 5	Upper Body Strength x 5	Legs Strength x 5	Upper Body Skills x 5	Full-Fledged Strength x 5
Week 6	V-Taper x 5	Legs Skills x 5	Frontal Strength x 5	Upper Body Strength x 5
Week 7	Core Skills x 5	Frontal Strength x 5	Legs Strength x 5	Upper Body Skills x 5
Week 8	Explosive Strength x 5	Frontal Strength x 5	Core Strength x 5	Frontal Strength x 5
Week 9	Legs Strength x 5	V-Taper x 5	Core Skills x 5	Full-Fledged Strength x 5
Week 10	Core Strength x 5	Upper Body Skills x 5	Core Strength x 5	Full-Fledged Strength x 5
Week 11	Legs Strength x 5	V-Taper x 5	Core Skills x 5	Upper Body Strength x 5
Week 12	Explosive Strength x 5	Core Strength x 5	V-Taper x 5	Frontal Strength x 5

CHAPTER 9: QUESTIONS AND ANSWERS

Tough times never last, but tough people do.

—*Robert H. Schuller*

I NEED TO LOSE FAT AND I WANT TO BUILD MUSCLE TOO. SHOULD I LOSE THE FAT FIRST BEFORE BUILDING MUSCLE OR CAN I DO BOTH AT THE SAME TIME?

It's a myth that you can't build muscle and lose fat at the same time. In an ideal world, it's best to get lean first then start building muscle by training hard and eating at a caloric surplus. The problem with that approach is, getting lean without strength training is incredibly difficult as creating a caloric deficit will get harder and harder as you get leaner.

The calories you burn during your training and the calories burned by the muscle mass you build will make it easier to lose fat. Follow the guidelines in the Diet Chapter to find out how many calories a day you should eat in order to train hard and lose fat at the same time.

WHY IS IT SO IMPORTANT TO KEEP A TRAINING JOURNAL?

Keeping a training journal accomplishes 2 things:

1. You get to know whether you are improving or not. You can't build muscle without progressive overload. You can tell whether you are improving or not by looking at your training journal and seeing whether you are scoring new personal bests (PB's) or not.
2. You get to know your weaknesses which you want to work on.

Use a timer to record how much time it takes you to complete a specific workout session. I track my workout sessions by the stopwatch function of the clock app on my smartphone. After I finish the workout, I note down the workout info on the notes app.

Besides keeping a training journal, I highly recommend keeping a diet journal to track your calories and macros. Moreover, take regular pictures of your body as it will motivate you to see your body improving.

I highly recommend you to regularly tape measure your waist, chest, shoulders, and legs. When your waist is shrinking and the other parts of your body are growing, you will know that you are on the right track.

WHAT IS THE CORRECT WAY TO BREATHE DURING THE WORKOUTS?

Exhale when you are exerting power and inhale during the negative portion of the exercise. For example, you will exhale when you are pulling in pull-ups or pushing in push-ups. Inhale during the negative portion.

WHAT DOES MUSCLE SORENESS INDICATE?

Muscle soreness indicates that you put an unusual stress on your muscles and they are trying to adapt. The workouts in this book are intense so muscle soreness is entirely expected, especially during the first weeks of your routine.

SHOULD I TRAIN WHEN I AM SORE?

If you are so sore that you can't even walk or lift a fork while you are eating, you should rest until the soreness regresses to tolerable levels. However, it's highly unlikely that you will be that sore. Soreness is expected especially in the beginning. If you can handle the basic movements, keep on training and the soreness will subside after a few weeks of training.

WHAT SHOULD I DO IF I CAN'T EVEN DO A SINGLE PULL-UP?

Proceed with the negative pull-ups and you should progress until you can finally do one and build up on that. Not being able to do a proper version of a particular exercise is never an excuse to not train. The easy versions of all the exercises are provided in the Exercises Chapter. Do the easy version until you can do the proper version.

I SEE ON THE INTERNET THAT THERE ARE HUNDREDS OF BODYWEIGHT EXERCISES BUT YOU ONLY INCLUDED 8. WHY?

The exercises in this book are the ones that will give you the most bang for your buck. They are simple and efficient. They don't consume your precious time. I believe that it's best to get done with your training in a few hours a week and mind the other parts of your life. The routines in this book will not eat up your time.

Moreover, simplicity makes it easier to stick to a training routine. Consistency is one of the most important parts of building a lean, muscular, and athletic body.

WHAT KIND OF SHOES SHOULD I

WEAR WHILE TRAINING?

If you are training at home, you don't have to wear shoes at all. All exercises are perfectly doable without shoes. If you are training outside or in a gym, flat sole shoes are more comfortable especially when you are doing squats where you should exert your body weight on your heels.

DO I NEED TO DO ADDITIONAL CARDIO TO LOSE WEIGHT?

No. High-intensity exercises will already work your cardiovascular system better than any other cardio workout. It's OK to do light exercise such as walking, swimming or riding a bike on your rest days for recovery purposes but none of it is mandatory.

WHAT ABOUT ACCESSORIES? DO I NEED ANY? SHOULD I USE GLOVES FOR PULL-UPS?

I don't use any accessories with bodyweight training so there's no accessory that I recommend.

I am not against using gloves while you are doing pull-ups although I don't use them. If your hands are hurting during pull-ups, nature will find a way to cover you up, which is to grow callouses in your palms. These callouses will come handy when one day you decide to lift weights. But, if want to use gloves, go ahead and use them. That's a tiny concern which will not have a significant effect on your results. What matters is the results, not what accessories you used while getting the results. Pull-ups with gloves produce the same gains as pull-ups without gloves.

DO I NEED SUPPLEMENTS?

I don't know any supplements that will give you a significant boost for losing fat or building muscle. Following the mindset and the diet guidelines in this book should be enough to get the best results.

That being said, I use fish oil and vitamin D semi-regularly but I am not sure whether they help or not. Creatine is said to provide a slight increase in training performance. I used creatine for a while and it positively affected my training performance but I am not sure whether it was a real or a placebo effect.

As a general rule, don't expect miracles from supplements.

DOES PROTEIN POWDER HELP?

Protein powder is good a way to get protein but if you are getting enough protein through your regular diet, you don't need it. If you are counting your macros and you are certain that there's no way you can meet your daily protein goals from your regular diet then it's probably a good idea to take protein powder.

SHOULD I WORRY ABOUT OVERTRAINING?

I've been training around the world for years and I've seen maybe 2 people that might be overtraining and that's a maybe. As you will be training 4 times a week with the training routines in this book, you don't need to worry about overtraining. There's plenty of time to recover.

MY MUSCLES/LUNGS FEEL LIKE THEY ARE BURNING DURING TRAINING. SHOULD I KEEP TRAINING ANYWAY?

Yes. The feeling of burning is expected with high-intensity training. It means that your body is adapting. The burning sensation will subside as you progress.

I FEEL PAIN DURING A PARTICULAR EXERCISE.

SHOULD I KEEP TRAINING ANYWAY?

Pain is a different story than burning. If your pain is preventing you from performing the exercises in proper form, yes you should stop training and see if the pain goes away after a few days of rest. If the pain persists, see a specialist.

HOW LONG WILL IT TAKE ME TO DO A PROPER PULL-UP/PUSH-UP/ETC.?

It depends on your body fat percentage and your starting level of strength.

You will progress if you keep on doing the easier version of the exercise and keep following the diet and training guidelines in this book.

AM I TOO OLD TO FOLLOW THE ROUTINES IN THIS BOOK?

No. I've heard the "I'm too old" excuse from people of all ages including some 18-year-olds.

I am 43 years old and I keep scoring PB's (personal bests) in my strength training workouts. You are not too old to train unless you have a terminal disease or a debilitating injury.

I DECIDED TO BUILD THE BEST BODY I CAN IN THE SHORTEST AMOUNT OF TIME POSSIBLE SO I AM DOING THE MAIN ROUTINE. BUT, THE WORKOUTS ARE TOO DIFFICULT. WILL THEY GET EASIER AS I PROGRESS?

Sure, they will not be as tough as at the beginning but I designed the workouts in a way that they will never get easy.

You will rather build the mental toughness to push through hardship.

Remember, if it gets too easy, you are not improving at all. Spare the easiness for the time when you are thoroughly content with your body and you are only training for maintenance. Maintenance is infinitely easier than progress. But first, you should get there by pushing through hardship. If you do it right, it will not take you a long time to achieve your physique goals.

I HEARD THAT ABS ARE MADE IN THE KITCHEN. IS THAT TRUE?

"Abs are made in the kitchen" is a lie that is told to the gullible masses who want to believe that they can get six pack abs without training hard. When these gullible people believe that they can have abs just by dieting, they will buy the diet products of the liars. That's a profitable lie for the people who tell it but not for the people who buy it.

If abs were made in the kitchen, every skinny person would walk around with six-pack abs which clearly is not the case.

Ab muscles are muscles too. If you want to grow your ab muscles, you must train them. If you don't expect to grow strong arms without training your arm muscles, you shouldn't expect to get six-pack abs without training your ab muscles.

Diet is only required to burn off the fat that is covering the ab muscles you build by training hard.

WILL I BUILD SIX-PACK ABS WITH THE ROUTINES IN THIS BOOK?

You will train your ab muscles intensively along with your other muscles. Having six-pack abs is about building the ab muscles and burning the belly fat covering those muscles. If you do your workouts and follow the diet guidelines in this book, you will get six-pack abs when you are down to 8-10% of body fat.

I COMPLETED THE 12-WEEK ROUTINE IN THE BOOK. WHAT DO I DO NEXT?

If you completed one of the beginner or intermediate routines, try completing the main routine.

If you completed the main routine and you are content with your physique, you can switch to maintenance mode where you train moderately to keep your shape.

If you believe that you have the potential to make further progress, you can repeat the routine for another 12 weeks.

If you are content with the physique you built by bodyweight training and you now want bigger muscles, you can switch to lifting weights. The foundation you built with the program in this book will be of tremendous help with your weightlifting.

I COMPLETED THE PROGRAM AND DOCUMENTED MY PROGRESS BY TAKING PICTURES AT THE BEGINNING AND THE END OF THE PROGRAM. I AM HAPPY WITH MY PROGRESS. WHAT SHOULD I DO?

You can send your results to contact@rippedwithbodyweight.com and I will publish them with your permission.

HOW CAN I CONTACT YOU IN CASE I HAVE FURTHER QUESTIONS OR ANY OTHER PROBLEMS?

You can contact me at contact@rippedwithbodyweight.com.

CAN YOU DO ME A FAVOR?

Thank you very much for buying and reading my book.

I'm confident that you're well on your way to building the lean and muscular body of your dream - provided that you follow the 12-week program outlined inside. But before you go, I have a small favor to ask...

Would you take 60 seconds and write a quick review about this book on Amazon?

Reviews are the best way for independent authors like me to get noticed, sell more books, and spread our message. I also read the reviews and utilize the feedback for future updates and books.

Click here to leave a review on Amazon.com

I appreciate your feedback and look forward to hearing what you have to say.

ABOUT THE AUTHOR

My name is Lane Goodwin.

I am the proprietor of LaneGoodwin.com.

My goal is to teach my readers how to be a great man.

I believe that every man should make self-improvement a lifelong goal.

I write about self-reliance, personal responsibility and discipline, masculinity, time-management, fitness, mindset and other topics which serve a man to build himself up to become the man he wants to be.

If you like this book, make sure to visit LaneGoodwin.com.

Also be sure to join my free newsletter to receive updates on new posts, books, and other stuff that I am working on.

MY OTHER BOOKS

How To Be A Superior Man

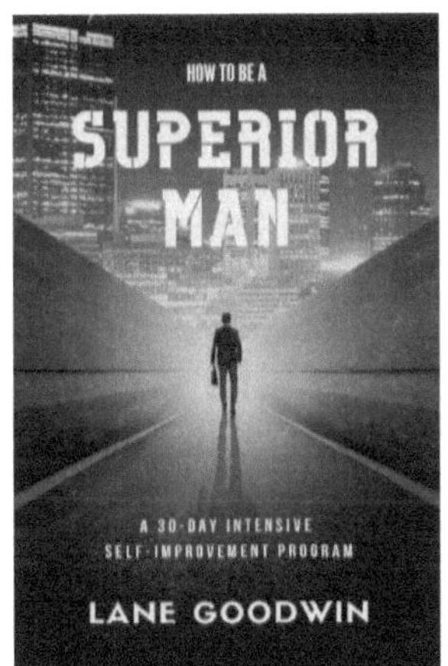

How to Be a Superior Man is an intensive self-improvement program to improve your life and your value as a man.

It provides an actionable plan which consists of the mindset principles, tools, and the relevant tasks you will perform for the next 30 days that will enable you to master yourself, take full control of your life and mold yourself into the man you want to be.

By the end of the program, you will emerge as a better man with better mental and physical strength, greater control over your life, and tangible results which will improve your self-belief and encourage you to achieve more. Click here to buy on Amazon.

www.ingramcontent.com/pod-product-compliance
Lightning Source LLC
Chambersburg PA
CBHW031254250726

48655CB00005B/2220